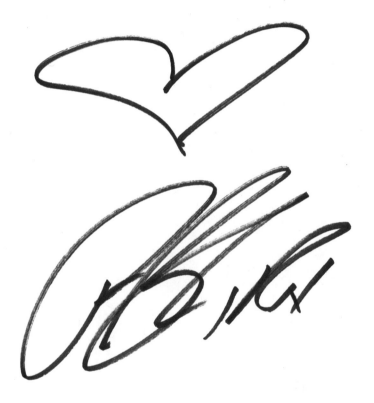

"Rich Bluni has done it again! In this book, he brings us right back to feeling great about our work. And he does it this time by encouraging all of us to connect to our work instead of focusing on the job. He moves us through each chapter by bringing us closer to our work, helping us realize the amount of self-worth we gain as we bring the artistry back to our occupations.

"All of us desperately need to read Rich's words of encouragement, inspiration, and engagement. Imagine a world where all of us were truly engaged in our work! This is the world Rich creates in the pages of this book. He helps us bring back the spirit of connecting and engaging in the amazing things we all do every day. He calls us to action in his style of sentiment mixed with humor and real-life examples.

"Anyone needing a lift, looking for a brighter workday, or searching to reconnect with feeling great about their profession needs to read this book. Fluffy stuff??? I would say fantastic stuff! Well done, Rich Bluni."
—**Liz Jazwiec, RN, Award-Winning Author and National Speaker**

"Once again, Rich shows us why he is one of the best. He'll make you laugh, cry, and, most of all, think. A master storyteller, Rich teaches through his own and others' experiences. A must-read for me and my entire team!"
—**David L. Callecod, FACHE, President/CEO, Lafayette General Health**

"In *Oh No...Not More of That Fluffy Stuff!*, Rich uses real-life stories that will hit close to home for everyone who reads this book. His valuable strategies that each of us can use today will improve how we view and

react to the people and world around us. A must-read for anyone looking for peace and engagement at work, at home, or in their personal lives."
—**Greg Paris, CEO, Monroe County Hospital & Clinics**

"This book provides the solution to current corporate culture woes that so many Fortune 100 companies face today: SELF-ACCOUNTABIL-ITY!!! An inspiring read and refreshing reminder that some things should never change!"
—**Gina Collins, Head of Entertainment Marketing, Coca-Cola North America**

"Rich has always been a brilliant presenter, connecting to the soul and emotion, the true levers of change. His new book does this again, in spades. It is funny, compelling, actionable, and challenging with practical, personal examples of life and work circumstances that all of us face every day. This book is the altar call of leadership! Rich has the unique ability to wrap teaching around personal connection and story and to distill those principles into leadership application to change ourselves and everyone around us."
—**Stephen Beeson, MD, Author of** *Practicing Excellence* **and** *Engaging Physicians*

"This book inspires us to not only change the world but to be the change we wish to see. It challenges us to reach deep within our own hearts so that we may impact the hearts of others."
—**Heather Long, MSN, BA, RN, Vice-President/Chief Nursing Officer, Florida Hospital Altamonte**

"Once again, Rich Bluni uses his insight into the everyday world of healthcare to help us connect not only to what matters most, but to *who* matters most...our coworkers, our patients, and ourselves! Use this book as a desktop reference to build your own engagement and that of those you are fortunate enough to call friends and coworkers. If you've heard Rich speak, reading this book will be like talking with him. If you haven't, look for the first opportunity to be in his audience. Rich's message, either spoken or written, has always left my bucket fuller than before."

—Dan Collard, Senior Leader, Studer Group

"This book offers practical and engaging insights into how to navigate and develop within one's professional and personal environment."

—Kathryn Keller, PhD, RN, Associate Professor of Nursing at Florida Atlantic University

Oh No...
Not More of That
Fluffy Stuff!

The Power of Engagement

Rich Bluni, RN

Published by:
Fire Starter Publishing
913 Gulf Breeze Parkway, Suite 6
Gulf Breeze, FL 32561
Phone: 850-934-1099
Fax: 850-934-1384
www.firestarterpublishing.com

ISBN: 978-1-6221800-2-8

Library of Congress Control Number: 2013937579

The stories in this book are true. However, names and identifying details have been changed to protect the privacy of all concerned.

Printed in the United States of America

DEDICATION

This book is dedicated to:

The three great loves of my life: my amazing wife, Dawn, and my two sons, Rhett and Luke. You are gifts from God, and I cherish and love each one of you with all of my heart. Your love sustains and strengthens me. I am blessed beyond words by you.

TABLE OF CONTENTS

FOREWORD

A Word from Quint Studer

I've always been a big fan of fluffy stuff (and I don't mean cotton candy and teddy bears, though they're nice, too!). I mean the kinds of things people call "soft skills"—qualities like having a positive attitude, working well with others, being able to resolve conflicts, saying please and thank you.

And I also mean the biggest soft skill of all—*caring*.

Think about it this way: The ability to insert a PICC line is a hard skill. The ability to insert the PICC line while making the tearful nine-year-old patient laugh despite the needle jabbing in her arm—*that's* a soft skill.

Realizing why it's important to make that little girl laugh—and choosing to approach every workplace interaction with that same level of sensitivity and thoughtfulness—is employee engagement.

It isn't just about how we deal with our patients, either. It's about how we deal with our leaders, our employees, our fellow team members. It's also about how we deal with *ourselves*—taking responsibility for the fears, shortcomings, bad moods, and bad habits that make us human.

Rich Bluni explains all of this beautifully in this book. I think you'll agree that his stories and insights really bring the subject of employee engagement to life. That's because he believes, and lives, his message every day. (If you've read his first book, *Inspired Nurse*, then you're already familiar with his compassion, his sense of humor, and his own deep engagement in his life's work. If you haven't, I'll just say you're in for a treat.)

I've known Rich for a long time. I've watched him grow as a speaker and pour his heart and soul into his message with a passion that's hard to describe. As a fellow speaker, I can tell when someone has really touched an audience. I've seen many people wiping away tears during one of his presentations.

All of this is my way of saying that Rich is the real deal. His authenticity shines through on every page. Somehow, whether he is speaking or writing, Rich is able to let down all of his defenses and give himself fully to listeners and readers. It's a real gift to be able to connect with others in such a powerful way.

Rich and I joke around a lot with each other. It's kind of the cornerstone of our relationship. I tease him, sometimes in public, about the huge following he has gained. Yet in all sincerity I know exactly *why* he has that following (besides the fact that he is so likable and relatable, I mean). This stuff is so important to people on a personal level, as well as to organizations that are trying to move the needle on results.

Rich says it over and over in this book (and in fact has been saying it for years), and I agree: Employee engagement is actually not a "soft" issue at all. It's a critical work skill wearing a fluffy disguise. It's actually a profoundly serious issue for two reasons: a) Engagement is in short supply, and b) It's deeply connected to outcomes.

It's easy to be an "endurer" or a complainer or just a person who coasts through the day with their eye on the clock and their mind on the weekend. (We all know someone like this, don't we?) In fact, a 2011 Gallup study showed that 71 percent of American workers are *not* engaged in their work.

That's a shame because there's plenty of evidence that engagement pays off. An article in the January 2012 issue of the *Harvard Business Review* shows a clear connection between employee engagement (here, described as "thriving") and an organization's bottom line. The study reported in "Creating Sustainable Performance," by Gretchen Spreitzer and Christine Porath, found that:

"...people who fit our description of thriving demonstrated 16 percent better overall performance (as reported by their managers) and 125 percent less burnout (self-reported) than their peers. They were 32 percent more committed to the organization and 46 percent more satisfied with their jobs. They also missed much less work and reported significantly fewer doctor visits, which meant healthcare savings and less lost time for the company."

Of course, in healthcare "the bottom line" isn't just about dollars. It's about saving lives, curing illnesses, and staying viable in order to serve even more patients in the future. We all know this. It's just that, sometimes, stress and negativity can overwhelm us, and we might forget—temporarily—that we know it. That's not good for our patients.

For all of these reasons, employee engagement is a hot-button issue for leaders in all industries in our global economy. It certainly matters to healthcare leaders who want to help their organization adapt quickly and effectively to intense, unrelenting change. But it *also* matters to individual employees.

Engagement is good for your career. It should be self-evident that people who throw their heart and soul and the full force of their intellect into their work are also incredibly sought-after employees.

In my experience, and as I discuss in *The Great Employee Handbook: Making Work and Life Better*, engaged employees are harder working and more resourceful than the clock-watching types. They're more innovative. They're more willing (and better equipped) to find solutions to their own problems.

They're better at collaboration and communication.

They're higher performers (and they attract other high performers to the organization).

What's more, they're happier and more fulfilled—not just at work but at home as well.

Yes, healthcare is tough and stressful. It's going to get even tougher and more stressful as time goes on. This is just a fact of life, and we can't change it. What we *can* change is how we choose to show up at work.

We can choose to be cynical and hurt ourselves, our organization, and our profession—or we can choose to find the passion and enthusiasm that makes our work worth doing.

It's hard to imagine anyone deliberately choosing the first way. I really believe that 99 percent of people want to choose the second way—but maybe they don't know how. If you're one of them, this book can help you change the outlook, the attitude, and the habits that are hurting you and those around you.

Read this book. Try some of the exercises. I think you'll find that your work life improves and so does your home life. And maybe you'll thank Rich Bluni for opening your eyes to a deeper, better, more meaningful way of approaching your journey.

By now it should be obvious that employee engagement is not passive. It's not something employers do *for* you. It's something you do for yourself. All employees at all levels (and yes, this includes the C-suite) need to take responsibility for their own success and happiness both in and out of the workplace.

When we do, we come to experience this thing we call *work* on a whole different level. We discover the richness, fulfillment, and meaning that have been there all along...and our lives are changed forever.

PREFACE

When you meet someone for the first time, one of the first questions you ask them is probably, "So, what do you do?" You ask that question because we are often defined by our "work." In fact, our "work" is a big part of how we see ourselves.

That's why it's so interesting that while we are very comfortable defining ourselves by our "work," we also seem to be at ease talking negatively about it. Think of the phrases you most often hear regarding work. Things like, "Another day, another dollar!"; "That's how they do us around here!"; "We're just the forgotten ones here in the basement!"; "Hey, I am just living the dream!"; "Can't wait for Friday!" And usually, that last one is said first thing Monday morning!

We define ourselves by the very thing we almost feel obligated to put down, our work. It's almost as if we've unconsciously been saying, "I dislike who I am." After all, if you're defining yourself by what you do, and yet you denigrate it, that's basically what is happening, right?

J-O-B VS. W-O-R-K

I wonder if we are a little confused about the difference between two commonly used words—"job" and "work." Think about your "job." It's all the stuff you *have* to do. It's the degrees and certifications you had to get. It's the skills you need. It's the amount of hours you work and the tasks and duties you have to complete. It's your job, and that's just the way it is.

Now think about the word "work." See, it seems to come from a different place. Think about an artist. They rarely call what they do their "job." You never hear someone say, "Michelangelo, he did a decent *job* painting that church ceiling in Italy!" No, what you probably will hear is, "The Sistine Chapel is one of Michelangelo's greatest *works!*"

Poets, authors, singers, actresses, and painters rarely define what they do as their "job." Of course, your job and the skills it requires are important. Artists, for example, need to have the tools of the trade and need to know how to use them. A painter must know how to hold her brush, how to mix paints, how to apply to the right medium. She must know her easel, her brushes. She must study and learn shading and lighting. In other words, she still needs to have the "job skills," but her satisfaction, her passion, comes from her connection to her work. That's where her heart is. That's where her spirit is.

LIGHTING THE MATCH: WHAT CAUSES BURNOUT?

A lot of us feel burned out on our jobs. Yet, paradoxically, burnout isn't really *about* our jobs. For example, I have never met anyone who overcame burnout by taking a certification class. Not a one. I believe we overcome burnout when we get in touch with our work. We have to connect back to our reason for being.

Most of you reading this are masters at your job. Many of you would probably even be considered experts at what you do. But I don't think job expertise insulates you from burnout. Based on my experience talking to literally tens of thousands of people, seeing their faces, and hearing their stories all over the U.S. and Canada, I don't think a lack of job skills is the leading cause of burnout. That's like saying the number one cause of divorce is that people don't know what to say at the wedding ceremony. I'm not buying that.

So if burnout doesn't come from lack of job skills, then where does it come from? I believe it comes from lack of engagement. And what *is* engagement? It's the sense of feeling tuned into, a part of, a contributor to our work, our mission. Engagement, in a sense, is the opposite of burnout. Where burnout is a separation from our work or our mission, engagement is a connection to it.

If we all can agree that most of us know our jobs pretty well, I am going to throw something else out there. I think most of you are pretty smart. I come from a healthcare background, and I know there are a lot of educated, knowledgeable, and highly trained individuals in that field. I am sure that most of the people you work with, for, and around are pretty bright too.

So, if we can agree that there is a lot of burnout on the job, that there is a need for engagement, and that there are a lot of intelligent people in our respective fields, what does that tell us? It tells us that if burnout could be solved *intellectually*, we would've figured it out a long time ago!

But what I hope you'll get out of reading this book is that the approach to fixing burnout comes from a deeper place.

It's not a drought of intellect that is causing all of this burnout. It's a drought of spirit. I think we are all like artists who know how to hold a brush but can't see a sunset in our imagination. So, we just sit looking at a blank canvas, wondering where the sunset is. We are singers who have excellent breath control and can read music accurately but can't find the heart to sing our song so we sit in silence. All the skills in the world, all the knowledge, won't bring you the joy of losing yourself in your work.

I want you, like a great artist, to have a masterpiece of a life. I want your work to be more than just a place you spend eight, or twelve, or four-teen hours! You spend so much time "on the job"—you've spent years and hours training for what you do—don't you deserve to feel some joy when you're doing it?

NOT JUST FLUFFY STUFF?

Is this all a bunch of "fluffy stuff"? I don't know. I think that's just what people who have given up say. After all, it is so much easier to be the sarcastic one making fun from the back of the class than the one putting themselves out there and taking a risk. I am asking you to take a risk. Come to the front of the class even if the "cool kids" are making fun of you.

After all, who cares? Understand that you will spend many years work-ing. What is it that you want to get from those years? Will your whole life just be punching a clock, sending out those silly Monday morning emails about wishing it were Friday? I hope not.

You have some choices to make, here and now. Choice One is to put this book down and walk away. If you do, you'll probably continue on with what you've been doing. Things may go up and they may go down, but, you reason, it is safer to go with what you know. You will get the results you always got doing what you've always done.

Choice Two is riskier. Keep reading. As you go, be honest with yourself. Take the chance that you may see yourself in a few of these chapters. You might laugh, you might (gasp!) cry…but unless you're too far gone, you will *feel something*. Wouldn't that be cool? You may also choose to *do something*. Even cooler. Then you may notice that you have *improved something*. Super cool! And then your work will *mean something*! Uber-crazy cool!

While I make you no promises and I hold for you no expectations, I do have a wish for you. My wish for you is that this book helps you along a path. There's a reason why you're holding it right now. My wish is that this book brings you closer to your work. My wish is that you go from seeing what you do as "making a living" to "living as you were meant to be."

I hope you see the work of art in what you do.

INTRODUCTION

SOMETHING FLUFFY THIS WAY COMES

He had a look on his face like he was smelling a rotten hamburger, long left behind, squished under a car seat on a hot July day. "You want me to do what?" he asked, making no attempt to hide his disdain. Clearly, this wasn't going to go very well.

I was coaching a "seasoned" CEO on ways to connect to his team. All I ever heard from this guy was how difficult it was for his team to "open up" to him and "be honest" and how "disengaged" they all were. I had to wonder how often he flashed his "smelly rotten hamburger face" at them. However, I wasn't sure saying that out loud would have much benefit. Instead I opted for another approach.

"Winston," (All names have been changed to protect the innocent, and not so innocent! Winston and his story are a combination of stories to protect privacy.) I began, "I think you need to not only think outside the box, you need to throw out the box completely. If you don't, you run the risk of getting the same old results over and over again. What could be the worst thing that would happen?" I asked, not really expecting an answer. But I got one anyway.

"They'll think I'm an idiot," he answered. *Okay. Do I fold?* I wondered. Nah. I'm not a fold kind of guy; I'm a "throw yourself all in" kind of guy.

"Okay, Winston, what's worse?" I asked. "They think you're coming from somewhere different, an idiot, as you would say, or they dread working for you because they don't see you as anything other than 'the boss'? And as a result they continue to avoid you and tiptoe around you?"

He looked at me. His face changed, ever so slightly—maybe not the "smelly rotten hamburger face" but more like smelly, slightly-older-than-you'd-want-to-eat asparagus face. Ah...progress.

"Go on," he said.

"Winston, you're an experienced leader," I told him. "You understand finance, goal-setting, and accountability. You were a CEO at an age when most people were still getting excited about getting their first business cards. But you've said yourself that you feel disconnected, unexcited, and less passionate about your job. You told me you sense that your direct reports and even frontline team members are feeling disconnected as well. You obviously care about the people you are leading.

"You're asking me to help you. I will. But, you're going to have to trust me and move out of your comfort zone. You're dismissing something before you've even attempted it. It is not going to kill you to try this. Please."

He took a long look at me. For one second it looked like he was going to refuse. He folded his hands. He inhaled. He closed his eyes. He spoke. "If one person laughs, if one person rolls their eyes, I will stop the exercise and I never want to hear about it again. Deal?"

I shook his hand and said, "Deal."

TAKING THE "FLUFFINESS" PLUNGE

The boardroom seemed quieter than usual. It had been a month since Winston and I had had our talk. Today was the day Winston would follow my suggestion. He took his seat. The leadership team all quieted down. Winston cleared his throat. I didn't know what he was going to say. He wanted this to be all him.

I have to admit, I had a moment of doubt. He seemed so tightly wound. *Would this work?* I wondered. He looked up. There was something about his look that captured everyone's attention. What was going through their minds?

He looked at his notes. He spoke.

"My mother died in my arms when I was in my twenties. I literally felt her take her last breath. It was like a sigh, and I remember that it blew my hair out of my eyes. It was more peaceful than what I had seen in movies and on TV. It felt instantly permanent. It was then that I knew I wanted to make a difference in the world. I wanted to make sure that no one ever came to a hospital fearful of the people working there.

"My mother had incredibly good and bad experiences. She came from a generation that both venerated and feared healthcare. I had been asked to leave the room prior to her passing by a hospital worker. I refused. That person called a manager. He asked me to leave. I refused. They called an administrator. He asked me to leave so that 'the people here can do their jobs.' I refused.

"I held my mother in my arms. They looked at me. I looked at them. We were enemies. On opposite sides. A nurse came in; in those days her title was 'head nurse.' She regarded the scene before her and looked at me over her black horn-rimmed glasses. She was the same age as my mother. The others stepped back and kind of looked at me like, 'Now he's gonna get it.'

"She said, 'I have a son your age. I love my son. He's out there fighting in Southeast Asia. He's as tough as his daddy was. I know that neither hell nor high water, much less some overbearing folks who have forgotten why they work in a hospital, could tear him away from me if I was at the end of my days. Any mother would hope the same of a boy she carried, and fussed over, whose bumps and bruises she kissed away and whose grades and choices she worried over. Why, it's the very least a son can do for a mother. You hold your mother. This is my department. What I say goes. Your momma would do the same for me if the shoe was on the other foot. I know she would as a mother. You hold your momma, Winston, you hold your momma...'

"With that, she shot a look towards the other two in the room that sent them scattering. It wasn't too long after that that my mother died in my arms. I never forgot that. And that is why I got into healthcare. I had never dreamed of being a hospital CEO. I wanted to run a factory, or lead a marketing team of a huge corporation. But, on that day, I knew I had to do this work.

"That's my story. I know everyone around this table has a story. I know that you all have different reasons to be doing what you're doing, and I think we need to share that. I didn't want to tell this story. I thought you all would laugh at me, or think maybe I'd gone soft. But then I realized something. I lost something. I lost that feeling I had when I got started. I had mastered my job, but I forgot about my work. Maybe in some ways I also lost you. I lost your respect, or maybe your loyalty.

"I don't want to be that guy standing in a room waving a rule book around trying to rip a dying mother out of her son's arms. I never want to be that guy. I wanted you to know that things are going to be different around here. I want to hear your stories. I want each of you to take a week and write it down, and we are going to get together for lunch and tell our stories. Then the next week after that, I want everyone to go around the room and tell each person at this table what you respect about and are grateful for about each person.

"I know this is different. But I also know that most of you are feeling a little burnt out these days. I can see it. I have an amazing team. I wouldn't trade any of you for anyone else. I don't want you to lose your passion for what we do. So, would you all be onboard with doing this?"

The room was silent. Not like slightly-lower-volume silent, but outer-space-floating-around-the-planet-Neptune silent. The chief nursing officer stood up. She was a brilliant woman. PhD. Smart. Articulate.

"All I have to say is thank you," she said. She put her hand on her heart. The chief operating officer stood up. He started clapping. The whole team stood up. They all started clapping. The CEO did something I rarely saw him do. He looked at me and he smiled. I smiled back.

He was smelling the roses now.

If I learned anything from that experience and the literally hundreds of others like it, it is that stories and gratitude can be amazing cures for burnout and waning passion for our work. Stories and the personal connections that they help create, along with gratitude, are the cornerstones of employee engagement. Whether in healthcare, industry, sales, marketing, ministry, or education, we've bought into a misdirected belief that getting "smarter" always leans to getting "better." While this is part of the equation, for sure, there is so much more to this.

Yes, Winston and his team followed through. Yes, things improved.

ROUNDING REALITY

If you're wondering what led to Winston's initial reluctance to follow through with what I was asking him to do, it began with a conversation about a topic that many leaders find a little mushy—rounding. "Rounding" is when a leader plays offense instead of defense. He asks questions of his team to assure they have what they need, to find out about their issues or concerns, and to see what he can do to help work them out.

One question leaders should ask when rounding is if there is anyone the employee feels should be recognized (praised, rewarded). This conversation also provides the leader with an opportunity to praise the person he/she is rounding on if there is reason to do so. What I learned from Winston is that he didn't want to do that part, saying, "I just need to make sure they've got the stuff they need. I don't want to get all personal with them."

And in fact, Winston certainly wasn't the first leader I had ever heard push back at that point in my conversation with them. Often, I would hear, "Oh no...not more of that fluffy stuff!" So in response, I always say, "You're telling me your team feels burnt out, unproductive, stuck in a rut like they've lost hope...but you're going to revive their spirit by making sure they understand the latest financial numbers, and maybe send them to a seminar on how to interpret the latest healthcare laws, and somehow THAT is going to fill their spirit?"

My question usually either causes a moment of silent reflection or a look of horror on their faces. But eventually there comes an acceptance of the absolutely undeniable truth that real change—organizationally, professionally, and certainly, personally—comes through connection, communication, spirit, encouraging others to connect to their *why*, and yes, being a little "fluffy."

JUST TRY IT

As you read *Oh No...Not More of That Fluffy Stuff!*, you're definitely going to come across topics that could be considered "touchy feely," "soft," "light," or "happy." *Fluffy*. (Hey, the title should have clued you in!) You might be a little resistant to these concepts at first, and that's okay. After all, ours is a society that often rewards the toughest, meanest, and most aggressive, at least initially. There is nothing wrong with being assertive, even aggressive, at times, in our work and life. Give me a goal and I will be assertive about making it happen. Bother someone I love and I will be aggressive about ensuring that you don't do it again. I'm sure you're similar.

But why can't we also be assertive about passion for our work? Why can't we be aggressive about pursuing peace in our lives? What if the energy, so often wasted on game playing, positioning, being passive-aggressive, worrying, being anxious, being afraid, and back-stabbing, was focused on being less judgmental, on being more forgiving, on communicating better, and other similar, much healthier attitudes and actions?

What if we were honest with ourselves? I mean really, really honest. Look at your work life. Could it be at least a little better? Yes. Of course it could be. Is it going to improve through luck and chance? Yes, that possibility exists. So does winning the Powerball Lottery, but I wouldn't depend upon that as your retirement plan.

Of course, making these positive changes will take some work and effort. You will like some of the concepts I point out, mostly because they may fit your present leadership belief system, and that's great. You won't like others. That could be because they don't fit your belief system, but I ask you to do something: Unless I suggest something that you believe is dangerous or an abomination and affront to all that is good and decent...just try it, okay? I promise you, there are no abominations. At least none that I am aware of!

THE JOURNEY AHEAD

What I want to do is make you think. Get you out of a rut. Help you to see that there is a better way. You *can* feel better. You *can* be more productive with your time. You *can* prosper. You *can* have an abundant, meaningful, beautiful work life. You probably wouldn't be reading this book if you didn't, on some level, at least "hope" for that. I, for one, am honored and grateful that you are reading this.

We are about to go on a journey, and I want to accomplish a few things. First, I want you to relate to what I discuss. I hope you see yourself and others in my stories, descriptions, and anecdotes. I may describe something and another person may pop into your mind. Pay attention. That's significant. It helps you to relate the concept to your present life situation.

You may recall an occurrence in your life and see how it could've gone differently. You may vividly see yourself, or hear your own voice. That's powerful, as I believe that is your very spirit talking to you. Listen to your gut. When you connect to a story, put the book down and let your thoughts take you on a ride. Write them down. As a society, we like to be told things rather than feel things. We are losing the ability to trust that sacred voice that comes from within. Don't lose that.

Second, I want to make you uncomfortable. (In fact, there's a whole chapter on this.) Being uncomfortable means we hit on something that you need to work on, and working through that discomfort is how you will grow.

Third I want you to take action. You have to do something! I'm not here to make you feel good. If you want to feel good, play with your kids or your dog. Get a massage. Eat some chocolate. Sure, you deserve to feel good, but that's not what this book is about. I want you to do work. Just like feeling sore after a tough workout, I want you to feel like you "worked out" your spirit. When I suggest writing something or saying something or trying something, it is not enough to think about it. You must do it. So, I want you to relate, feel uncomfortable, and take action.

One last caveat. This book is no substitution for professional or therapeutic help. I'm not a therapist. I don't pretend to be, but I love and appreciate those who are. There are certainly some awesome ones out there. If you are struggling with depression, anxiety, anger, addiction, or the like, seek these folks out. The suggestions I make in this book are to get you to think. Not to diagnose or treat you. I'm just another regular person like you. I'm just a "friend" who wants you to get to a better place in your work. Just like you would go to a dentist for a toothache without hesitation, you should seek counseling for "heartache" without hesitation. (Unless your heartache is more like actual chest pain—then please call 911!) But seriously, take care of yourself. Promise?

So now comes the good stuff (or the fluffy stuff, if you will). Are you up for it? I know you are!

CHAPTER

1

HERE COMES THE JUDGE...

When you look for the good...you'll see things as they should be, you'll *be seen differently, and you will find more than meets the eye.*

Are you judgmental? No? *Really?* Well, here's a reality check—yes, you are. It's okay. Unless you're reading this aloud as part of group therapy, no one needs to know that you thought you were judgment free.

Let's face it, we judge. We really do. A lot. Like, all of the time. In my talks, I often recommend an exercise I call "Whatcha Thinkin'?" Here's how it goes:

Next time you're at work, I want you to try an experiment that will show you how much you judge. As you start your day, I want you to be very conscious of each person you encounter, especially your colleagues, at your place of work. If you get in an elevator with them, sit next to them in a meeting, help them to do something, or even pass them as you walk by, if you work with this person and you know them even a little, I want you to be very purposeful about finding/thinking/recalling one GOOD thing about the person.

It can be *anything* good—a trait, a behavior, a recent kindness you observed. Anything. And as you try to do that, I want you to catch your first thought and maybe even the second. (I find that by the third thought you are already self-correcting yourself and have focused yourself on pulling up the good thought.) Basically, become very aware of the first couple of things that pop into your head as you try to think of something good about that person. You might be dismayed to see how "not good" these first impressions really are.

Following are some first-thought examples that were recently shared with me by a dozen or so people who tried this exercise:

1. Wow, he gained weight.
2. I hate when she does that stupid wink thing.
3. There is NO good in him.
4. I am so glad she transferred.
5. Please don't talk to me. Please don't talk to me. Please don't talk to me.
6. She really needs a mint.
7. I can't believe he never apologized for that obnoxious email.
8. I bet it physically hurts her to smile.
9. Does he actually own a mirror?
10. Jerk.
11. I'd be smiling too if I never had to do real work.
12. Oh, great, "The Fonz" is giving me the "thumbs-up" again.

See a pattern? The funniest thing is, as you just read these you had some thoughts of your own. Like, *How rude!*; *What a shallow person!*; *I never think things like that!*; *Who's "The Fonz"?* You get the idea. We have become so judgmental that we even judge people for judging.

I'm not saying we are all horrible people, who will eventually end up beating someone up on a reality TV show, but what I would suggest is that these thought processes can be, at the very least, adjusted. When you do this exercise, I think you will find that even when you are trying to find the good in someone, you have a default mode of thinking. And usually it takes you to a judgmental thought, a recall of a grudge, or a past offense.

WHERE DO YOUR JUDGMENTS LEAD?

Let me be honest. I don't know if we can ever be 100 percent "judgment free" or that we'd want to be. I mean, if you're walking down a dark alley and a guy is walking towards you wearing a hockey mask and carrying a bloody ax, it's probably okay if you judge him and make some basic decisions based on that. For example, you may want to run in the other direction.

In fact, maybe it's built into our human makeup to judge, like a survival thing. Maybe some caveman named Krog looked at another of his clan and said, "Wow, Krug ate a lot more of that wooly mammoth than I did. That's not fair. He always does that..." And from that moment on, every time Krog and Krug put down their clubs and gathered around the cave fire to share some spicy pterodactyl wings with the clan, dirty looks and disapproving grunts were exchanged. I'm sure even Neanderthals had the capacity for sarcasm!

So, you wonder, what happens after I spend the whole day noticing my judgmental thoughts? Will I end up curled up in the fetal position in my cubicle after realizing how mean I am? Well, don't do that, first of all. What I'd want you to do (preferably sitting in a chair and not in the fetal position) is reflect on your day. Ask yourself these questions, and if you can, write down your answers:

1. How did that go for me?
2. What were the first thoughts I had as I looked upon a colleague?
3. Do I hold grudges? If yes...why?
4. If I made a habit of finding the good in others, what would change?
5. Why would I NOT find value or wisdom from this?
6. Would I want to say out loud the first thought I had about each person to them?

Here's what I and many others have learned from this experiment: Our default is not usually leaning towards what is good in another person. I don't know why. And frankly, I'm not as concerned with the "why" side of the equation. The point of the exercise is that it cries out to us to just "do" something.

So, when looking at Frank, the sarcastic guy who always looks like he's about to offer a mocking comment and who seems to always be the first person in a meeting to point out your mistakes in front of your boss and your boss's boss, I want you to dig deep. When you see him, for a moment look past his flaws and notice something good...maybe his shoes are always polished, or he always has a pen to offer when you forget one, or he always speaks so proudly of his daughter. There is always *something*.

I truly believe the "Franks," or whoever elses of the world, are put here to remind us that in every situation, every challenge, every difficult relationship there is a bigger lesson. There is a wake-up call, a moment of reflection, an opportunity to see the good in people. In each other.

Can this exercise teach you something about yourself? You can be the judge of that.

CHAPTER
2

PSYCHIC VAMPIRES

*Challenging people can exert enormous pressure upon us,
sort of like the pressure of the earth upon the rocks below.
It is up to us whether we allow it to make us crumble or to
turn us into a gem.*

Psychic vampires are not the cool, sexy, brooding vampires we read about or see in movies. They don't have fangs. They're not any better looking than the rest of us. They can walk around in the light of day and probably love garlic bread.

Psychic vampires don't suck blood...they suck the energy, joy, life, and happiness from the room. Often, simply with their mere presence. You know exactly the kinds of folks I'm talking about.

When you have to spend time around a psychic vampire, you always leave feeling drained and exhausted. Your mood darkens. Your energy level decreases. You have the strong urge to take a nap.

Most psychic vampires have perfected their skills. For them, sucking the joy, life, and happiness from a room is a power play. They know that if they can be negative and draining enough they will get their way because no one else will have the energy to fight back. They don't need to overpower you or get in your face. They simply wait until your eyes are half closed and your head is dropping. Then they strike! Kind of like a python that slowly strangles its prey until the soon-to-be-meal is so weak it offers no resistance to being consumed whole. Got the picture?

STEP AWAY FROM YOUR PITCHFORK

Psychic vampires walk among us. Oh yes. And while you may fantasize about gathering the other villagers together with pitchforks and torches to march upon their cubicles and flush them out of the office, that probably won't go over well. HR usually looks down upon bringing pitchforks into the workplace (unless you work on a farm!), but for most of us that approach just won't bring positive results. So how *do* you vanquish the psychic vampire threat? Here are a few ideas:

Stop talking about them to others. When you gather with colleagues in dark hallways, break rooms, and at lunch tables to talk in hushed voices about "Darth Vera in Finance," you're feeding the proverbial blood to the psychic vampire in your life.

You're giving her strength and power. You're giving her a scary mystique that will influence your coworkers who don't have to work closely with Darth Vera. Of course, she doesn't possess any real magical powers. And she is no more powerful than the rest of you.

So, the first step is to stop the gossip. Don't feed into their myth. They are probably much weaker and afraid than you can even begin to imagine. In fact, some of them might actually be pretty good, deep down. (Remember Winston in Chapter 1?) It is highly likely that their behavior masks deep insecurity. Once you stop feeding that insecurity, you can begin to break through to the real person.

Call 'em out. Like a playground bully, once someone is actually brave enough to stand up to them, psychic vampires will back down. So, when your resident PV makes a sarcastic comment about something your peer has just suggested during a staff a meeting, simply say, "Rhonda, respect is important in this organization. It's listed as number one in our organizational values and standards. When you roll your eyes and laugh at one of your colleagues, you are also mocking our values. I'm uncomfortable with that."

Keep in mind this is not the time to start bringing up past transgressions. Stay focused on the here and now. Use a calm voice. Connect her behavior to the "big picture." Bringing up the company's "values and standards" or mission statement is a great way to do so.

A good friend of mine tried this approach with great success. Practically word for word. After he said those words in a meeting, there was silence. My boss took the reins and said, "I agree. We have to be comfortable with being able to talk openly as leaders. If anyone disagrees, I'd like that person to be transparent and respectful about it. Is that clear?" Nods all around...well, except for the death eyes darting out from the PV.

But, after the meeting, the PV did not follow through with her usual post-meeting tear down. She seemed somewhat humbled. She retreated to her lair. All seemed quiet in Transylvania that night.

One quick sidenote: PVs have mastered the art of stealth. They know how to eye roll, mutter, laugh, and shoot dirty looks while still remaining invisible to their leaders. As a result, their behavior is often not as obvious to the "boss" in the room as it is to those who are on the receiving end. So don't always expect the "boss" to know that this goes on.

Try a little love. Okay, this probably seems out of place given the suggestions you've read so far, but it is another tool to have at your disposal. Many PVs' bad behavior is a defense mechanism. They've developed their PV persona in order to make up for other weaknesses in their character.

Most of them were not the most well liked or popular kids. What they may have lacked in brains and/or personality, they made up for with sharp responses and an uncanny ability to sniff out the weak and prey upon them. What they've had little of is friendship and kindness.

When I was a teenager, I went through a short time when I had some success and popularity, and a few jealous "mean kids" set out to make my life miserable. And they did. The used the usual teen stuff—rumors, threatening notes on my car windshield, the random midnight toilet papering of my yard.

And while I was blessed to have great friends, who were genuinely happy for me, the bullying I experienced at the hands of these other kids was like the end of the world to me. One day, my mom saw how unhappy I was and asked about it. We talked and she gave me the best advice: "Kill 'em with kindness." And so I did. I went out of my way to compliment the kids when it made sense to do so. One day, one of them was about to get beat up in a schoolyard scuffle, and I stepped in on his side. He looked shocked. He actually asked, "Why did you stick up for me?" I just shrugged and said, "I hate seeing someone getting picked on."

Another kid was falsely accused by a teacher of doing something, and I went to the vice principal's office and offered witness testimony for the defense. I vouched for his innocence. He was saved from being expelled and kicked off a team. So out of the five who were out to get me, three of them became very good friends and we made amends. One backed off and kept his distance, and one remained in the "I hate Rich camp." Those odds were pretty good. Not perfect, but good.

It was a great life lesson. Of course, there is an art to it. First of all, you don't want to make it your goal to "cure" the PV. That's not a good use of your energy. Secondly, you don't want to come across as a pathetic kiss-up. Just look for opportunities to compliment or manage up something they did or said. If you do it right in front of the PV, chances are you will see a "What's she up to?" look on their face. Just go with it. If it happens when they are not around, it will get back to them.

Most likely they will not come to you with freshly baked muffins, give you a hug, and repent of their past sins, but here's what does happen: They'll see that you are taking the high road. And they're savvy enough to know that if they keep taking shots at you they will look like morons and will lose what little influence they have. So they'll back off. Or... your behavior just might light that little spark of humanity that still exists deep down within them causing them to truly come around.

Either way you have nothing to lose. It is a win-win. From a PR standpoint, you look good and show your maturity and kindness. It is always the stronger person who chooses the kind route. Also, you show the PV that you don't fear them, and you open up the possibility for a PV to reform.

CHAPTER

3

BE COMFORTABLE WITH BEING UNCOMFORTABLE

To get to that, you gotta go through this!

He was in pain and staring at a family portrait on the wall across from him. What a warrior. I was visiting a friend, a young father who had been injured in a bike accident. He was recovering from tremendous orthopedic injuries and was inspirational in his work ethic and pain tolerance. His physical therapist was putting him through the paces.

He nodded at me without losing his focus on the portrait hanging on the distant wall. It was a photo of his wife, his young son, and him on bicycles on a sunny day. He was squinting as he looked at it, so I assumed he was having difficulty seeing it. I got up, ever the helpful dude, and plucked the picture off the wall so that he could see it up close.

"No! Put it back!" he yelled through the pain of his therapy. "I'm just moving it closer so you don't strain your eyes out of their sockets!" I explained. He stopped his exercise and put his hand up to tell the PT they were taking a break.

"Rich, I want to keep it far away because it reminds me of the truth."

"What truth?" I asked.

"The truth that me getting back on a bike and riding a marathon is something I *will* do, but there's a lot of work that has to be done between now and then. I put that picture barely within sight so that I can remember that I have to get to that," he pointed strongly at the picture on the distant wall. "I gotta get through this!"—he motioned to the strengthening device he was using. "That's reality, man. To get to where I want to be, where I will be, I've got to work hard. I've got to hurt. I have to push through it. If I think my goal is closer than it really is, I will get lazy. I can't afford that."

I carry those words with me everywhere. I even have them tattooed across my back. (Okay, not really.) "To get to that. You got to get through this." That doesn't sound too easy. That doesn't sound too comfortable. Most of us would rather believe, "To get to that, I need to ease into this...find a shortcut...then, take a break...then, try again later. Maybe after all that, I'll have a nap and some cocoa." Nope. Sorry, that won't cut it.

We don't like being uncomfortable. We hate it so much that we even try to trick ourselves into thinking that we are comfortable. Case in point: the snooze button on the alarm clock. It's all a ruse to play the "I'm comfortable" game. Let's say you need to get up at 6:00 a.m. So you set the alarm for 5:50 a.m. so that you can hit the five-minute snooze button a couple of times, supposedly "fooling" yourself into thinking you snuck in a little more sleep. Wouldn't it make more sense to get the 10 minutes more of actual sleep and simply set the alarm for 6:00 a.m.?

Being comfortable with being uncomfortable is a way of disabling the "snooze button" on your life and deciding that from now on you're going to jump right up and face the day. This is a concept that pertains to any area of your life that requires improvement, change, or progress. Want to get a higher degree? Then, you'll have to save up to cover the tuition, stay in instead of going out with your friends, miss your cousin's destination wedding in Bali, prepare to write papers rather than watch your favorite TV shows. You will be uncomfortable and you best get used to it until you are holding that diploma in your hand.

Want to get fit? It is going to be uncomfortable. You'll need to eat salads instead of Snickers bars and go to the gym instead of the new cupcake bakery after work. (I love cupcakes. Just wanted to put that out there.) You'll be sore. It will hurt to stand up. It will hurt to sit down. (Anyone who has ever done an intense leg or lower body workout can attest to the fact that for about 48 hours, they avoided having to sit on the toilet for as long as humanly possible, secondary to how painful it was to plant their bottom on a hard toilet seat.) But if you want to get in shape, if you want to sport bulging biceps, shapely toned legs, and a six-pack set of abs, you will need to get used to a lot of discomfort.

Professional confrontation is a little like that as well. While there have been entire books written on how to confront an issue or have a conversation that may be uncomfortable, the basic concepts are somewhat, and surprisingly, simple. Relationships require uncomfortable conversations and decisions; being a parent, a leader, a good friend, a teacher, a good spouse, or significant other all require the discipline of being comfortable with being uncomfortable.

What positive habit, discipline, or behavior are you a little "uncomfortable" with? For example, does the idea of telling someone that they did a great job make you feel goofy and silly? If so, that's a huge sign that you need to throw yourself into getting comfortable with being uncomfortable. Usually when you say, "I'm just not like that," or, "That's not me," understand that you're making a false statement. The real statement should probably be, "I don't like doing that," or, "That's not something I want to do right now."

Who we are, for the most part, is a choice. Sure, it's a little more complex than that. Our backgrounds, our upbringings, our parents, etc. all play a role in how we develop. But when you drill down, for the most part, we *decide* what and who we are.

And while you have no control over the weather, what another person is about to say or do, or if your favorite sports team goes to the championship, you DO have control over what you think about. So, when you say, "I'm uncomfortable with complimenting my staff/team/friends/ bodyguard/personal chef/wife/boyfriend/kids/probation officer/German Shepherd," what's really going on is that perhaps you've decided that doing so is uncomfortable and you are avoiding doing it so that you can avoid the discomfort. Well, here's some news for you: Just like you choose to "buy into" this set of beliefs, you can choose to "buy out of it."

Following are a few common areas of "discomfort" and what you can do to get comfortable with them.

1. Communication. Breakdowns in communication can quickly get you into trouble. In healthcare, for example, the number one reason for major errors or sentinel events is usually attributed to some breakdown in communication. Of course in life one of the main reasons for divorce or break-ups is poor or incorrect communication.

Why does communication cause us so many problems? Well, usually it leans toward the negative. Don't believe me? Okay, when's the last time you complained about the service at a restaurant, criticized your spouse, or moaned about an annoying client? You've probably done at least one of those things or something similar in the recent past. Comparatively, how many times recently have you asked to see the manager to rave about the server, praised your spouse for one of their accomplishments, or told a client or coworker what a pleasure it is to work with them? While you may do these things some of the time, they certainly aren't the norm for most of us.

Through repetition we've conditioned ourselves to be more comfortable with corrective communication than complimentary communication. Ever been in a relationship where the majority of what was said to you was pointing out your "issues"? What you were wearing, what you said, your appearance, what you should've bought for a birthday gift? Stinks, huh?

How weird that many of us feel more comfortable correcting than complimenting. If you self-assess and find that you are one of those folks who "feel weird" complimenting or thanking others, then immerse yourself in this advice: Revel in your discomfort. Bungee jump into the bottomless abyss of happy talk! Too much? Okay, here are a few tips:

a. *Make a concerted effort to compliment three people a day.*
   Putting this into action utilizes one of the many gifts of the human brain: habits. Habits, of course, can help and hurt you. Some are good. Some are bad. Some can kill you! They're powerful things.

Unfortunately, it seems these days many of us have gotten into the habit of pointing out flaws. We love to watch the shows where the primary source of entertainment is watching people who can sing, cook, design clothes, and so on much better than most of us get eviscerated by judges. Judging has become part of our culture. We criticize for entertainment. But, of course, it's not fun for the person on the receiving end.

Better habits start from repetition. Three a day—that's all it takes! You could compliment the barista who made a great mocha for you, your spouse for shoveling the snow so you could get out of the driveway, and the volunteer for wearing a sharp-looking tie. These all count.

Yet many of us worry that when we compliment someone they will wonder what we are up to or that we will sound like we are "trying too hard to be nice." That kills me! We actually worry people will accuse of us of trying too hard to be nice but we AREN'T afraid that people might think we are trying too hard to be mean? What the? Three compliments a day, every day. Minimum. You're doing a great job! (That was one of mine; two more to go!)

b. *Don't be afraid of thank-you notes.* They're like taking compliments to the next level. They're like mini contracts of good feelings that you sign and give to another person. Keep a few in your car, purse, backpack, and so on to unleash on unsuspecting members of society.

    If you have an amazingly kind bank teller, leave her a note. (Just be careful with bank tellers. Usually when they're handed notes at work it goes in a *whole* other direction!) Had a great server? Leave him a thank-you note and maybe a few extra dollars. Did your daughter's teacher make a difference and inspire her to learn more about science, creating an excited sparkle in her eyes? Then send a thank-you note to that teacher. (Teachers deserve as much appreciation as we can give!)

Once you have the notes in reach, it will amaze you how obvious it is to see all the people who are out there conspiring to make your life a little nicer. It may feel weird and very much uncomfortable at first to hand the always-nice and fast-working barista at your coffee shop a thank-you note. But trust me, the look on his face and the occasional free muffin or extra shot of espresso, which I always interpret as being told I'm on the right track, make it very much worth your while.

Of course, it goes without saying that you shouldn't get into the business of handing out thank-you notes simply because you might get something out of it. What I think you'll find, though, is that you get something out of it every time because it feels so good to show someone your appreciation for a job well done.

c. *Make it personal, too.* Let's get personal for a second. I know this is all about work, but we are more than that. When's the last time you told someone you love how much you appreciate them? Your teenage son might have emptied the dishwasher without being asked (yes, I've heard it happens), your spouse or loved one may make your cup of coffee every morning with just the right amount of sugar and creamer, your best friend may have recently sent you a very funny email that made you smile on a morning when a smile did not seem to be in the cards. Tell them how much you appreciate those gestures. This may be uncomfortable at first. Your loved one may even think you're up to something. Good, it will add spice to your relationship! (If you ARE up to something, please stop it; you're going to get caught!) Or maybe you're at odds with them over something, and it would be uncomfortable to be the first one to break the ice.

Just do it! We create so much unnecessary misery for ourselves jockeying for position. At the end of your life, do you want someone who loves you to stand over your deathbed and say, "Well, we had 1,342 arguments during the many years we were together, and you won 934 of them! You win! Go in peace!" (If you answered "yes," I love you for your honesty, but you need help ASAP!) At the end of the day, it really isn't all that important who wins and loses arguments in your relationships. So, even if you're still mad that your loved one forgot to take out the garbage (again) last week...get over it!

So, what should you say? Use simple, direct words. For example, "It really means so much to me that you always make my coffee in the morning. I feel very loved when you do that." It's that simple. And if this is not your normal way of communicating, those words will not only stop your loved one in their tracks, it may cause them to make complimenting a habit as well.

I'm sure some of you are rolling your eyes right now. (Be careful! My mom used to tell me they could get stuck like that!)

But, come on, somewhere deep inside that heart of yours you know it would feel good to have all of your good deeds and achievements pointed out to you. NOTHING bad can come of this. A well-placed compliment can change a rut. Those words can make a kid feel valued. They can lead to a reciprocal communication, which may lead to things just being a little better in your world.

What's the worst that can happen? Okay, they may blow it off, or roll their eyes, or even make fun of you. But that's just because they aren't used to being complimented. Just do it and keep doing it. Around the fifth time you compliment someone, it will begin to feel "normal."

And yes, if you don't have a chance to tell someone the compliment, you can always write it on a note and stick it in a backpack, lunchbox, briefcase, purse, or jacket pocket for your loved one. We have allowed the art of the "love note" to disappear. Revive it in your life.

Yes, it starts at home, but the good feelings won't end when you walk through the doors of your workplace. Your home life absolutely affects your work and vice versa. It is worth the discomfort. Trust me.

What I hope you've learned here is that the first step to embracing being "uncomfortable" is related to communication. Whether it's with our colleagues at work, our loved ones, or random members of society, compliment, appreciate, acknowledge, and verbally "hug" those who share your life. Do it until it becomes "who you are."

2. Trust. This is a biggie for most of us, and especially for you higher-performers. We have a difficult time trusting our coworkers enough to be comfortable with delegating and sharing responsibility. When faced with an overflowing workload, we often just say, "Never mind...I'll take care of it all." Why? Because at some point in your career, you probably gave up some aspect of a project or assignment to someone else and they dropped the ball, leaving you holding the bag. So now you trust no one. Unfortunately, that attitude doesn't usually lead you to success; it usually leads to burnout.

Here's something to try: Think of one project, duty, or responsibility for which you are presently the sole "owner." Could be a budget, a client project, or a charity fundraiser. Reach out to some of your teammates and delegate aspects of the project. Ask your leader to help assign some components to others in order for you to be able to ensure success. If only it were that easy, right? Of course, if you're a control freak or have been wronged by doing this in the past, just the thought of delegating important tasks makes you uncomfortable. Good. Now, do it anyway.

Sure, it may mean having an uncomfortable conversation with your boss or colleague, but we've already learned that getting comfortable with being uncomfortable with certain aspects of communication is an essential part of creating a more satisfying work life.

3. Solutions. For those of you who are leaders (formally by title or otherwise), stop allowing people to bring you only problems. Start encouraging people to bring you solutions, too. Often leaders are expected to be *lifeguards* instead of *swimming instructors*. Here's what I mean: Every time a staff member comes to you and says, "Somebody needs to do something about this!" don't respond like a lifeguard by jumping in to save them. Instead, be a swimming instructor. Teach them to swim.

Respond with, "I agree, this is a problem (insert *dramatic pause* here). Now, what do *you* think should be done about it?"

Asking that question accomplishes something big. It helps train that person to solve problems rather than just report them. It takes very little effort and/or intellect to point out a problem. How many people do you come across who always seem to know "generally" what's *wrong* in the world? They say things like, "They never get this stuff right!"; "Why can't these guys get it together?"; "Doesn't anybody care around here?" But rarely do these folks attempt to offer an actual solution.

In addition to creating problem solvers, you teach yourself not to rescue, but instead to coach and teach. As bright as you are, you don't have all of the answers. If you think you do, or others think you do, you are setting yourself and them up for disappointment. You're also heading for burnout.

Many on your team have great ideas, but perhaps they lack the initiative, the confidence, or the comfort to speak up. Perhaps they've been conditioned to just bring it to "the boss" (whether you are a leader with a title or not) so that you will figure it out. Instead of "carrying the burden" as the chief workplace martyr, ask those with issues and complaints to come to you whenever they feel they must, but insist that they bring with them a solution.

Be direct. Tell your team that you trust their minds and creativity. Tell them that you know that they are able, intelligent, and resourceful people and that you want them to be a part of each solution. This will serve two purposes. It will serve notice to the "PVs," who like to throw bombs simply to incite unrest, that this type of behavior is not welcomed in the organization's culture.

"Complaining" is for the weak and powerless; "collaborating" is for the strong and powerful. Make this an unavoidable message that is declared from the mountaintops! The PVs will learn very quickly that the old way is not going to fly. The other purpose asking for solutions serves is the creation of ownership. If the "team" collaborates and is a direct part of a change, they will support that change. They will drive the implementation and they will ensure that everyone does the same.

Have you ever wanted to have or create something and "convinced" the other person it was *their* idea? Then all of a sudden the doors opened and all was well in your world? It's kind of the same psychology, and it works for those above us or alongside us. If I feel a sense of "this is mine," whether it's an idea or an object, I will protect it and I will advance it.

So instead of you always being the one to "present the solution," allow them to be the architects and the drivers of it all. This is how you harvest intellectual capital and create an environment of engagement and subsequently growth.

4. Self-Assessment. I believe that we get something a little backwards sometimes. I am a big believer in creating and writing down goals. You're reading this book because I followed through with the exercise of writing down a specific goal and then ensured that my actions, thoughts, and meditations lined up with creating this book.

Goals are the locked door that we must open to make our "stuff" happen. But, of course, a locked door needs a key. I believe the "key" is self-assessment. Often we set goals and come up with action plans *before we self-assess*. It's fine to set a goal, even a lofty one, for which to strive. Most people don't even get that far. If you write down your goals and follow their progress even irregularly, you are far ahead of the norm. So what I'm proposing may be a little surprising. I think before we set those goals, we first have to *know thyself.* Where to begin? Let's take a look:

1. Who are you, to you?
2. Who are you, to others?
3. What do you think you're good at?
4. Need to work on?
5. What do people around you see that perhaps you don't see?
6. What are your strengths?
7. Your weaknesses?
8. How do you personally define these words: Success, Failure, Happiness, Sadness, Love, Passion, Prosperity, Beauty, Power, Spirit, Inspiration?
9. Do you like what you "see" in the mirror?
10. What's the biggest "win" of your life?
11. What's some "unfinished business" in your life that you'd like to finish?
12. Where do you feel you "failed"?
13. When are you most joyful?
14. What does "fun" mean to you?

Of course, there are tons of other questions you could ask yourself. Don't be afraid to dig deep. As a wise teacher once told me, "*Harass your spirit.*" In other words, make yourself uncomfortable!

Be brutally honest with yourself. What's the worst that can happen? If you know deep down that your temper was the reason for your last break-up, even though you've been spreading the story around your circle that it was "just not meant to be," be honest enough to admit it was your temper even if it's just to yourself. Because if your temper ruined one relationship, rest assured it will ruin another one.

If you know, deep down, that your first impression of someone was wrong, admit to yourself that you need to be less judgmental and give people a fair shake. In fact, in general, we should all get more comfortable with saying, "I was wrong." You have to be honest with yourself before you can ever dream of having real, honest goals.

And of course, fruitful self-assessments are easier said than done. Start with spending some time alone. Write a list of questions like what I've shared and expand it on your own. Do a deep self-review. Unless you are a truly delusional person (and some of us are), you will have some type of breakthrough.

This is a very uncomfortable process. For some of us, it is like opening Pandora's box, at least at first. But if you can get through the discomfort, you will be impressed with who you become.

Take your time with it. Don't spend less than a week on it, preferably more. The amount of time and energy you put into it will directly correlate with what you get out of it. (Isn't that a universal truth for most things?) You may start off thinking getting to know yourself sounds like a fluffy concept, but I promise you there ain't no fluff in that stuff!

This can get pretty "heady." Basically you are asking the deep question, "Who am I?" There have been volumes written on this subject. It's one of those questions that has both easy and complicated answers. But at the end of the day, I would challenge that this is ultimately the question we have to ask if we want to live at a higher level.

And we certainly need to have a firm grasp of who we are if we're going to be able to be more connected to our work. I don't know who you are, but I know who you're not. You are not your degrees, your name, your history, your family tree, your title, your color, your gender, your salary, what someone told you you were, or your alma mater. These are all part of your existence but not who you are. People who have a strong sense of "self" are the people we love to be around, spend time with, and work with.

5. Talking about yourself with others. As you get more comfortable with self-assessment, you can take the next step, which is talking with others about yourself. This is a great opportunity to talk with a counselor or therapist. If you have issues such as addiction, past abuse, depression, or the like, please seek someone with the skills to help you. These professionals are often great life coaches. They can give you exercises, refer you to groups, or recommend books to read. Don't be afraid of this at all. Or you might be more comfortable seeking spiritual counsel from a trusted pastor, rabbi, or the like. Wonderful. Beautiful. Go for it! It can all be part of getting to know yourself! Certainly, trusted friends are also a great resource. Most of us have at least one friend who tells it like it is. They really nail the truth about us every time. Tough love is still *love*, and they may help you make some realizations you wouldn't have come to on your own.

Being comfortable with being uncomfortable is hard work. But that work will light the flame inside of you. Friction creates heat. Like rubbing sticks together. This work will light your fire. The largest candle in the world is no good without a wick. It's just a tower of wax. You need to light that flame.

CHAPTER

4

FORGIVENESS

It has been said that holding a grudge is like drinking poison and expecting the other person to die. I would tell you that forgiveness is like filling the other person's pockets with diamonds...but you become wealthy.

Sometimes people at work do messed up things. They lie. They are unkind. They gossip. Some people even go out of their way to hurt others. I'm sure you're nodding your head in agreement right now. Maybe you even yelled out a "True that!" That's how prevalent this behavior is. We've all experienced it from our coworkers at some point.

I don't care if you are in the highest levels of corporate importance, on a construction site, in a law office, in an ICU, or whether you're a nurse, a physician, a student, or a dog walker, if you work with other humans, there will be interpersonal conflict. Period. And conflict is the number one reason people struggle with their level of inspiration and passion for work.

However, let me start out by saying, for the record, sometimes that is a cop-out. Sorry. Sometimes it is easier to say, "I could be more inspired at work if THEY weren't all so difficult!" I can't tell you how many times I've coached an organization and had sit-downs with folks who would get very specific about how Martin and Sandra were IMPOSSIBLE to work with. Then I would sit down with Martin and Sandra and...you guessed it...hear the same complaints about the others! So, let's be really, really real. There are times when every single one of us could wear a shirt to work that reads "difficult to work with" across the front.

That being said, perception is often at least our reality, so conflicts do happen. In the workplace you have people from some diverse backgrounds who argue, problem solve, speak, and think differently. Sometimes those factors contribute to conflict. Sometimes it results from being competitive. Sometimes it happens because the organization has a culture that needs some work. Sometimes people are just mean. But what this all boils down to is this: Conflict happens! No matter how it is created or manifested, no matter what its "deeper" source is, in the end there is one sure-fire way to dilute it's power—forgiveness!

Forgiveness is a subject that can be quite controversial. I believe it directly contributes to our level of passion for life, work, and everything else. When you are carrying grudges or even outright hatred and disdain for anyone you are around, it changes the "air." You "vibrate" differently. People feel it.

Have you ever walked into a room where there were two people who despised each other, and even in the absence of yelling, rude comments, or visible signs of aggression, the tension in the air still feels so thick you could cut it with a knife? There's something to that. You feel it in your bones. It is an almost primitive reaction. No one has to say a word but you know it. You think, *Uh-oh, it's about to get ugly in here. I better get out before these two start throwing down!*

For small violations, forgiveness is easy. But it becomes harder as the perceived attack grows in magnitude. Forgiving a friend for scratching your car with their fender when they pulled out is easy. Forgiving the same friend for running over your dog in your driveway because they were on their cell phone is harder. Forgiveness could easily have been included in the Chapter 3 discussion on how to get comfortable with being uncomfortable, but I think it's so important that it needs a home of its own.

When I posted a comment about forgiveness on my Inspired Nurse Facebook page, it garnered the most comments and "likes" I had seen in awhile. It also received a few harsh comments. At first, I felt bad about those. Then, I thought more about the subject and realized that many people have been on the receiving end of horrific betrayal, hurt, abuse, lies, and backstabbing. Telling them to just "go forgive" is too simplistic and maybe even somewhat disingenuous.

I get it. There are people and situations that I've had to "forgive" because it was really hurting only me to not do so. In my own experience, far from it being a holy act of altruism, at times, forgiving has been purely about survival. I'm just being honest.

Personally, my faith drives me. You may or may not have a specific faith or "belief system" so I want to be as universal as possible with one caveat. Way, way, way smarter people than me have talked about and analyzed forgiveness. I'm trying to offer only a small peek at how I see it affecting our level of passion for our work and lives. It is a complicated and, for some, deeply rooted concept. And truthfully, I can only hope to scratch the surface. (Please re-read the last three sentences five times!)

Seriously, I'm treading on somewhat "sacred" ground, or maybe it's more like a minefield, but I'm willing to take the risk as I feel it may get you thinking. That's all. So, are we cool? Good. Join me for a walk into the minefield of forgiveness.

WATCH YOUR STEP

The pushback some of us feel towards forgiveness is that it means "forgetting" what happened and going back to how things were before. With apologies to any who might disagree with me for what I am about to say, I believe that approach could often be somewhat detrimental and maybe even dangerous.

But before we go there, let's establish that forgiveness is an act of "spirit." Forgiveness happens when you accept another's imperfection and move past or through a real or perceived shortcoming, error, hurt, or insult. It is when you choose to no longer feel anger or resentment towards someone for something they said or didn't say, did or didn't do.

It can be internally demonstrated. Meaning you can choose to forgive someone who may or may not know you've forgiven them. For example, they may be dead and gone, but in order to move on in your life, you forgive them. It can also be externally manifested. For example, I might ask you to forgive me for losing your passport, which I was supposed to carry, leaving you stuck in the country of Whatanastastan, famous only for its llama milk and rock throwing festivals. So, you feel forgiveness and then tell me *out loud* that you forgive me. Thanks, that was very nice of you!

So that's kind of a quick view of forgiveness from the internal and external points of view. There is some argument as to whether or not you "have" to forgive someone even if they didn't ask for it. In researching that question, I found that the answer varies based upon culture, religion, and background. For this conversation, I want to work from the assumption that forgiveness is something that you are doing for yourself, at the very least, so the much-hoped-for apology may or may not have been delivered.

Okay, so we've more or less "defined" forgiveness and/or allowed you to decide for yourself how you "define" it and how you understand the concept. Now, it's time to take a look at the "forgetting" part of the equation.

FORGET ABOUT IT?

Let's say you have a friend who lives with you. He has a significant addiction issue that he has not sought help for. And when you began sharing the apartment, you didn't realize how significant the addiction was. Okay, so, let's say your friend is powerfully addicted to collecting Elvis memorabilia. You come home one day and all of your valuables have been stolen by him and sold so that he can purchase one of Elvis's jumpsuits from an auction on eBay.

Your jewelry, TV, DVD player, Coach purse(s), and every other valuable thing you own are gone. The two of you have it out. He then tries to get some of your stuff back but to no avail. He says he's sorry. He even offers to let you try on the jumpsuit. He asks for your forgiveness. Let's say you love your friend and you forgive him. You choose to forget about the whole thing and pretend it never happened.

Two weeks later, he gets the PIN to your savings account, takes most of the money out, and buys one of Elvis's old guitars. Same old thing, he's sorry. You forgive him. In this case, would it be wise to forget again? Should you continue to live with him? Allow him access to your possessions? Assume that it's not going to happen again? I would say that would be most unwise. Do you agree? You do? Thank you, thank you very much. Elvis has left the building.

So, while forgiveness may be wonderfully applied, you probably should have the discernment to change or even end your affiliation with this friend, at least until he gets some help and demonstrates that his life is turned around. If you don't, you risk more loss and being taken advantage of.

You see similar events play out with families dealing with true addiction issues. They reach a point where they tell the loved one that they love them, but if they don't get help the family will no longer give them a place to stay, money, etc. Tough love.

So this is where a lot of people get hung up. They want to forgive and stop dwelling on the issue, but they feel they cannot forget, as it may open them up to continued harm. If a neighbor saw your dog walker beating your dog, even if you forgave them, would you continue having that person walk your dog? Chances are you love your dog enough to be unwilling to test the person's level of recovery. You might choose not to forget and instead protect your dog.

So, for our work, I would encourage you to forgive, but the forget part is somewhat optional and certainly situation-specific. I don't want you brushing past forgiveness because you think that it means you must still go back to how things were prior to the event. So forgive, but you may not necessarily always forget.

THE FORGIVENESS WORKOUT

Here is a little work for you to do. I recommend that you spend time thinking through these questions before filling in your answers.

1. Think about someone you have had, or presently are in, conflict with. Maybe someone at work took credit for something you did, or maybe you found out they have been repeatedly speaking very unkindly about you. I want you to ask the following questions of yourself. Feel free to write your answers down here or use a journal or pad of paper to expand upon them.

    a. What emotions do I feel when I see this person or hear their voice or their name mentioned? _____

    _____

    _____

    b. What do I feel physically when I see them, hear them, or hear their name mentioned? (stomach cramps, headache, muscle tightness, etc.) _____

    _____

    _____

    c. Are any of the emotions or physical manifestations I listed above healthy for me? Or, do they feel good or enjoyable? _____

    _____

    _____

d.   Has this person apologized to me? _____

_____

e.   If not, would it make a difference if they did? _____

_____

f.   Do I want to stop feeling and thinking in the ways listed in "a" and/or "b"? _____

_____

g.   Do I believe that this person is as uncomfortable/stressed/unhappy as I am about this situation, or are they going about life untouched by this? _____

_____

_____

What you may notice is that how you are feeling, both in your mind and body, is not good for you. When you look at that person or hear their name, your stomach goes into knots or tears form in your eyes, but I can almost guarantee you that that person is looking at you across their cubicle and all they're thinking is, *I wonder if I should wear a sweater tomorrow.* Most likely, they couldn't care less about how you feel.

In some ways, you're holding a grudge. You have not forgiven and you can't move on. I've heard it said that holding a grudge is like drinking poison and expecting the other person to die! Answering the questions I provided helps you self-evaluate and shed light on the whole thing.

Betrayal and hurt are dark stuff. But darkness cannot exist in the presence of light. Go into a pitch-black room and turn on a flashlight. The room has changed. So, by looking at this situation by answering my earlier questions, you get real and you change the circumstance. Now you can move onto the forgiveness part, and to be sure, there are a lot of ways to go about doing it. Here are some options:

1. Directly address and confront the person. Respectfully and calmly present your impressions and feelings about the issue. Let them know you're doing this with the hope that at minimum you can reach common ground and at maximum (if this is possible) you can reconcile the situation.

   Now, remember, as mentioned in my previous examples, you may not want or feel safe having a "reconciliation." It really is optional, and you have to determine if that is the right choice for you.

2. If you don't feel safe or wise confronting them, but you're tired of feeling like you do, write them a letter and express your anger, hurt, and confusion in detail. When you're done, sit quietly and re-read your letter. Say a prayer, meditate, and listen to your inner voice.

   Now release what you are feeling by tearing up the letter, burning it in the fireplace, or putting it into the shredder in your office. This approach provides two results. First, it allows you to get your thoughts out. To see them. To allow yourself to process what you're going through. Second, it allows you to be done with it. To forgive and to give yourself permission to move on.

3. Get with a trusted friend *who is not involved or part of the group associated with the person you are struggling with.*

Someone you trust who has no dog in the fight. Vent to them. Let it out. Tell them what this person did, how you feel, what you've been experiencing. Let them know your goal is to achieve forgiveness and freedom. They don't have to offer advice; you just need them to listen.

4. If you follow a religious or spiritual path and have a trusted advisor on the same path, then seek guidance through those beliefs or directly from your advisor. Your use and understanding of forgiveness may be strongly rooted in this path or belief system and it may even teach you differently from what you're reading here. Please, by all means, honor who you are and what you believe. Trust your heart and your gut.

5. And of course, if you are really struggling, or the issue is something like present or past abuse, threats, bullying, or the like, seek professional help. ASAP.

So your path to forgiveness may actually be made up of many roads. You may have a better idea than what I proposed, or yours could utilize a few paths. Maybe you feel it is safe to confront the person but first you want to write out your thoughts and then talk to your pastor, rabbi, invisible friend Harvey, or the village shaman. By all means, do what you feel is best. Maybe you want to write out your thoughts and read them to a trusted friend and then bury it under a tree in your backyard. Go for it. You know what works best for you.

Forgiveness is a direct way to uncover and reconnect to your passion. It is also a tool to knock away the barriers to your passion. Whenever you want to accomplish something, there are obstacles. Maybe you want to run the Boston Marathon but presently you get winded walking from your car to the Krispy Kreme shop. That's an obstacle. You need to remove the obstacle to achieving your goal by doing some work. In this case, training and exercising as well as changing your diet.

Carrying grudges and pain around is an obstacle to feeling empowered and passionate. It is poison to your soul, and I would say that there is some information out there that suggests being angry and bitter and holding grudges is probably also poison to your health.

My words on forgiveness should just be the beginning of your thoughts on the topic. Trust me, forgiveness is a beautiful and life-changing concept. There is so much more to it than I could possibly hope to address here.

In full disclosure, I am a work in progress as it relates to forgiveness. (Sometimes a little bit more "work" than "progress"!) But I am committed to ensuring that it is a cornerstone of who I am.

Read about it. Study it. Look it up. Ask about it. Look for movies or books with forgiveness as the theme. Take a class on it. Get a group of like-minded friends or even colleagues to talk about it. Look for examples of where it is lacking and ask yourself what you would do in those situations. Sometimes seeing how not to do something offers as many lessons as learning how to do it.

To paraphrase the late Jim Rohn, an amazing thinker and author, a formal education will make you a living but self-education will make you a fortune. That "fortune," I believe is more than just monetary. Learning about a subject such as forgiveness through your own reading and research can bring only value and worth into your life, personal relationships, and work relationships. I'm opening the door, but the rest is up to you!

CHAPTER

5

GIVE PEACE A CHANCE

The distance between pain and peace is measured between your ears.

Don't worry. Be happy. Oh, if only it were that simple. But, in some ways, it really is that simple. At least in theory.

Many people might agree that they aren't feeling a sense of passion for their work because at some level they do not feel a sense of peace. Usually feeling connected, passionate, and even inspired comes about because we have some level of contentment, grounding, or peace. In other words, you feel safe.

Many of us don't work (or live) in obviously "peaceful" places. Some may be in an actual battlefield because you are in the military and are stationed in a dangerous environment. For others, your workplace might just feel like a battlefield because it's full of "hostiles" who may not physically attack you but instead throw daggers with their eyes or use their razor-sharp tongues to slice you down.

Then again, you may work with amazing people, but the nature of your work puts you in contact with very difficult, trying, depressing, or stressful situations. Either way, and wherever you are, creating some peace for yourself is an essential step toward regaining or maintaining a sense of passion for what you are doing.

I have to be honest here. I think most people take on "victim energy" when the talk of "peace" comes about. What I mean by that is they decide to believe that a lack of peace is solely attributed and owned by "someone else." Rarely do people look in the mirror and admit, "It's ME!" (Psychic vampires have an especially hard time with looking in the mirror as apparently vampires don't have reflections!)

Remember what I said earlier about being honest with your "self." At the end of the day (or night if you're on night shift!), a lack of peace may be connected to external factors, but ultimately it ends with you. Unless the powers that be are going to pick up your workplace and move it to a "nice" neighborhood, give intensive therapy to every grumpy coworker/customer/patient/friend whom you encounter, or protect you in some way from encountering tough situations—none of which is likely to happen—it comes down to you. Only you. It was always *you*.

You have to first have some level of commitment or desire for encountering peace. You can't be a really angry person and just go out into the woods and yell out to the clouds, "I need some peace NOW!" Won't work. You will only frighten the wildlife. Might even get attacked by a raccoon.

You have to take some steps to align with peace. Decide what peace means as it relates to you and your world. Understand and believe that in order to have peace...wait for it...you need to figure out how to be peaceful!

GET ON THE PEACE TRAIN

Here's the secret. Peace does not occur *around* you, per se, it comes from *within* you. You can be on a mountaintop surrounded by natural beauty with the wind blowing gently, smelling the rising scent of lavender from the valley below, with gentle wind chimes serenading you along with birdsong and STILL not be peaceful if you aren't in tune from within. *The radio station can send the signal, but if you don't have batteries in your radio you can't dance to the music.*

You can work to change the world around you, and we all should do our part to make it a more peaceful and loving place, but no matter what, a true sense of peace will be something that you first choose to have, then work at, and finally commit to maintain. As always, be real with yourself. Ask these questions and take a few minutes to think through or write down the answers:

1. What does it mean to be "peaceful"? Is it more physical for you? Emotional? Mental? When you're not peaceful, or the least peaceful, what is going on? What do you see as a cause of this? What are you thinking or feeling?
2. Have you ever felt peaceful for a period of time? If so, what were you doing? What kind of people were you with? Where were you? Do you think the circumstances were more significant than what was happening inside you? How did your body feel? What were you thinking about? Talking about? What were your habits at the time as far as eating, sleeping, drinking, and working?

3. Who is the most peaceful person you know? What do they do? How do they speak? What is their demeanor? What do they talk about? What kind of people do they surround themselves with? Are they peaceful no matter where they are and who they're with? (Do you see that their "peace" comes more from within them or from outside them?)

4. Do you believe that you can achieve at least long moments or periods of peace?

5. Do you exercise? Pray? Meditate? Do yoga? Eat more of a "fast" or a "fresh" diet? How much water do you drink? How much sleep are you getting?

6. What kind of movies/TV/books/sports/music do you spend your time immersed in? Comedy? Horror? Romance? Action? Violent? Loud? Angry? Fast?

7. Do you spend any time walking in or being a part of nature? Hanging in a park, surfing, swimming, boating, hiking, walking your dog, throwing a ball with your kids?

8. When (and if) you get a break at work, what do you spend most of your time doing? Eating? Socializing? Gossiping? Surfing the web? Phone calls/texting? Getting your personal work done like paying bills, scheduling appointments, etc.? Reading? Listening to music? Meditating? Doing some spiritual work on yourself?

9. What do you think is your biggest external obstacle to peace?

10. What is your biggest internal obstacle to peace?

11. Now be honest...between questions 9 and 10...which can you truly and directly impact the most?

I can't answer any of these questions for you. I have a strong hunch of what your answer is for number 11. But beyond that, I can make assumptions based only on what I believe to be true and from what I've seen work in my own life and for others who "get" that you can't feel inspired and connected at work (or in life) if you aren't able to have moments of peace.

PEACE OUT...OR PEACE *IN*?

I want to give you some work to do. This will be very individual but hopefully meaningful. You won't be able to do it, though, if you haven't answered the earlier questions. So if you are skipping ahead and thinking to yourself, *I will keep reading and get back to this later...* BUSTED! Stop right now and please spend time going through the 11 questions. Be honest and real with yourself. When you've done that, and only then, please read on for your next assignment. (Isn't this fun!)

Let's get started:

1. Think about the peaceful people in your life. If there is one you feel comfortable talking to on a personal level, interview them. Ask them about peace. Ask them what they do to stay peaceful. Have they always been a "peacekeeper"? Or did they get peaceful after something tough happened to them? (I find the most peaceful people sometimes have had some real trials and challenges that, for lack of a better word, forced them into becoming peaceful.) What are their habits? Their practices? After talking with this person, see if you can model their behaviors. As weird as it may sound, even mimicking their physical movements can help you get closer to peace. The simple point here is to learn from a peaceful person. Find a peacefulness mentor.

2. Sit down in a quiet place and relax. Breathe deeply and slowly. Still your mind. Feel your body relax. Once you feel relaxed, picture a real life "unpeaceful" moment at work as it happened in the past. Choose something that stressed you out and that resulted in your reacting angrily or negatively or in a way that just felt bad. Run it through your mind as if it were really happening. Picture what others said and did. What you said and did. Just as an athlete will visualize a race before she runs it, visualization can help you get through your stressful moment. Picture the fight or problem as it really happened. If you lost it, yelled at someone, cried, said something mean, or walked away with your stomach in knots, whatever it was, mentally go back to that place. If you do this well, and it could take some practice, you will likely feel something physical. You may relive similar emotions and feelings. In other words, your head may hurt and you may have an increased heart rate. You may feel angry all over again.

    It is fairly common knowledge that the body often cannot distinguish between something actually happening or being thought about in detail. That's why when you think about someone you're very attracted to or love, even when they are far away, you may have a physical reaction. Your face gets flushed, blood pressure increases, etc. Even though they aren't there actually rubbing your feet (wouldn't a foot massage be nice?), your physical self reacts to them as if they were, just because you are picturing them so vividly. The same holds true for someone you strongly dislike. The mere mention of their name or the sound of their voice can create physical reactions.

Once you've reenacted this not-so-peaceful event as it happened, I want you to try something. Relax. Picture the exact same event, but this time, and this will take full use of your creative imagination, I want you to change the story significantly. Picture yourself reacting to the situation very differently. Instead of losing it, you are calm and still. Instead of reacting angrily, you feel compassion and maybe even love and forgiveness for the person yelling at you or criticizing you. Instead of chaos breaking out all around, people seem to handle themselves differently. They are now reacting to your peace and they are much calmer and even helpful and supportive.

You see yourself being calm. You have the whole situation under control. You feel what you would feel when you know, deep down, everything will work out for the best. Basically you are taking the out-of-control event that negatively impacted you and you are now changing the story so that you see yourself handling it gracefully and peacefully.

Yes, this is completely pretend. It didn't happen that way at all. But I know you can do this. Think about it. How many times have you totally exaggerated a story or a conversation to fit your argument or needs? Be honest, you know you have.

We all have the ability to use our imagination, and this is a powerful exercise for a few reasons. When we have been through something, sometimes in the moment we don't handle it the best possible way and we torture ourselves with "should haves." The power in this exercise is when you do it meaningfully, you may find when a similar event pops up the next time, you will seem to handle it more in the "perfected" way than you will in the real way from your past. Even if you saw only a 10 percent improvement, isn't that better than repeating the whole mess?

Most likely, unless you have your own reality TV show, you do not have cameras recording your every move and word. You are most likely also not an NFL player and don't have recordings of the "plays" you've done at work. But if you did, you would have the luxury of watching and learning from your past behavior just as athletes watch game film to improve their performance. These athletes understand that to be excellent at something it pays to not only practice on the field but also in their heads. Since you may not be able to invest in a film crew, you can achieve virtually the same results through the power of imagination.

After you have changed the story and "run the play" perfectly in your head, come out of your relaxed dream state and check yourself. How do you feel now? Maybe you saw something about that situation that you hadn't noticed before. Maybe you saw that there was "another way." Even though some people were acting like outright fools, maybe you noticed that you could have, at the very least, changed how *you* acted. Maybe in the "improved" version, you didn't take the name-calling personally. Instead, you felt sorry for the person who needed approval so much they repackaged your idea to look like their own.

Maybe you saw that you could have leaned this way, turned your head that way, or carried the ball closer to your body, figuratively speaking (well, unless you are an NFL player reading this...). You could at least, through the power of your mind, experience what it would be like to be peaceful in a challenging situation. This not only helps you deal with stuff that happened, but it also prepares you to do better the next time.

Peace takes work. You have to want this enough to be willing to sit in your chair and "run the play" in your head.

Some additional thoughts: If you find that you keep sticking with the bad outcome and get all flustered, stop and try again later. You may have picked something so overwhelming that it will take more practice. If that is the case, you may want to start with a less intense event first and work your way up to the other one.

You will find from this exercise that you possess within you more answers than you even realize. When I did this, I was amazed what came up for me. I saw someone who looked and sounded like me but handled things much differently. I found that when the same event happened again, I was prepared for it. It was like I had done a fire drill, and when I smelled smoke for real, I knew exactly where the exits were. I dropped and rolled and stayed down where the clean air was and I didn't get burned!

CHAPTER

6

IT REALLY IS BETTER TO GIVE...

Work is essentially a gift—of your time, your knowledge, your abilities, and your spirit. When done right, our work gives so much more to us than we give to those we serve.

When working on oneself, it is easy to get so focused on "self" that we forget that there is a whole world out there. You get so focused on "self-improvement" that you can go way overboard staying in your own little world... You think, *I need to do what I need to do for me!*

A lot can be said for taking time for self-improvement. But I do want you to consider the other side of the self-improvement coin, and that is that it is also essential to go outside your "self" and take time for others. When you do, I think you'll find that one of the best ways to feel more passionate about work and life is to make it one of your disciplines to give to others.

Giving comes in all sorts of colors. I want to suggest a few things that you can do and then I want you to think of some of your own.

Give money. For some people, this is one of the easiest ways to give. And of course, there are many ways to do it. Perhaps you can take some of your earnings and earmark them for a particular charity that resonates with you. If you like children, then maybe donating some money to a charity that helps children with cancer or one that helps homeless children is the way to go. Love animals? Then donate to a charity that protects endangered species. Worried about a particular cause or group of people? Then give some money that helps support that cause or lifts up those people.

Really, the choices are almost endless, even if your savings are not. You will run out of money way before you run out of charitable giving options. You may give from your surplus or as Mother Theresa used to say, "Give until it hurts."

Another great way to put money aside for giving is to reallocate the funds you spend on the little luxuries in your life. For example, take the money you spend on that double mocha-caramel-peppermint-iced-extra-whip latte every day, save it for a few weeks, and then donate it. Maybe the idea of making a little personal sacrifice like that one clicks with you and that's great. Maybe you would rather eat your shoes than give up your coffee and that's fine too. It doesn't matter where the money comes from as long as it is yours and as long as you're not accumulating debt or harming yourself or those who depend on you by giving it.

I actually had a friend who would work one or two overtime shifts per year with the intent of donating the money she made from those shifts to her charity of choice! Pretty cool. She said that it always seemed like those particular shifts were some of the smoothest work days she had. So, donate away.

Give time. Perhaps you don't have extra Benjamins, Jacksons, or even Washingtons flowing out of your pockets, and donating money is not an option for you. But maybe you have extra time. If that's the case, you may choose to give your time instead.

Opportunities to do so are everywhere. Help build homes for the needy. Volunteer at a soup kitchen. Help an elderly neighbor by doing some yard work for her. Fundraise for a walk-a-thon or bake sale. Usually these cost next to nothing and really require only your time.

Or think about it this way: At work there are probably tremendous opportunities for you to give your time beyond just checking off tasks on your to-do list. For example, there is probably at least one person on your team who is newer and perhaps could use some mentoring. Or maybe one of your colleagues always struggles with their budget, and you can do it with your calculator tied behind your back. Reach out to them and offer to help teach them how to do it. Let your coworkers know you are all about their success.

I believe a good leader says, "Look what I've accomplished," but a great leader says, "Look who I've helped become accomplished." Be a great leader. Help someone to be the best they possibly can.

Now, these first two giving options don't really require any "special" skills, but what can you do if you DO have special skills? Read on.

Give time—part two. Are you good at math? Writing? Know a lot about world history? What if you took that knowledge and did more with it than winning trivia night at a local bar? There are so many kids out there who need mentors. Tons of young people could use some help understanding a variety of subjects from algebra to adjectives to Abraham Lincoln (and those are just the "A" words I could think of!).

Volunteering to tutor young people is great, but keep in mind too, that there are also plenty of adults who could benefit from your expertise. Had some success in business? If so, volunteering to assist struggling business owners or providing some guidance to folks interested in your field would be something you could do. If you're in healthcare, go on a medical mission trip or volunteer at free clinics.

I know personally how rewarding medical mission trips can be. When I went on one to Honduras, what I found amazing was that even though I was doing the same things I did "at work" to get paid, it felt so much more rewarding and fulfilling doing it for free to help someone! Shocking. (And no, I never told my boss that!)

You can give your time and skill in "formal" ways like tutoring or mentoring, but there are also less formal ways to do so. For example, let's say you're a culinary wizard. Your niece has just graduated from college, she'll soon be living on her own, and you know she is less than skilled in the cooking department. Invite her over for a couple of cooking lessons and show her how with little cost, time, and effort she can eat healthy and well. After all, you know what they say: Give a man/woman a fish and you feed them for a day; teach them how to glaze, season, bake, and create sides for the fish and you feed them for a lifetime! Get creative. These opportunities are abundant.

Give your stuff. If you have a shirt in your closet that you haven't worn in seven years, chances are you won't be wearing it in seven more years. If your kids are in elementary school and you know you will not be having any more babies, but you still have a stroller or highchair sitting around, maybe you won't be using those things, either. If there are books that you have sitting around that are not bound in leather and etched in gold, printed by Benjamin Franklin or signed by Shakespeare, then perhaps you won't be reading them again.

What I'm getting at is that like most people, you have accumulated stuff. Some really good stuff maybe, but "stuff" nonetheless. You have clothes, toys, books, furniture, tools, and whatever else sitting around gathering dust. Spend some time and clean house! There are so many people, organizations, and charities that could find a home for your Barry Manilow concert t-shirt. I promise you.

I had a friend who decided that he was going to learn about carpentry. He had way more money than commitment or time, so he bought a whole lot of great tools— hammers, saws, clamps, gadgets, etc. He had pretty much everything you need to open up a carpentry business. He took a few classes, built a pretty decent birdhouse and then a doghouse. (No, he didn't have a dog. It was just easier than building a greenhouse!) Then he never touched his tools again until he moved them to the outside shed after his wife converted his woodshop back into the TV room. (Actually, it would be more accurate to say she "reconverted" it back to being the TV room while he was at work. He didn't notice for two days...yeah, he was a regular Mr. Fix It!)

But something really great happened as a result. Even though he lost interest in woodworking, he was always the most generous guy and he loved to give. He was at the grocery store and the young lady at the register was ringing up his food when her young husband came in with their little two-year-old in tow. He was just bringing their son in to give mommy a kiss. She apologized to my friend as she paused to kiss the little boy. While he waited, he overheard the young husband say he had good news as he had been hired to do some extra carpentry work. The young man said that even though he had to rent and borrow a few tools, there would still be a little left over for them.

My friend almost jumped on the poor kid! He politely interrupted and asked the young man what he did for a living and what tools he needed. He found out that the couple was struggling between going to school, working two jobs, and taking care of their son. He also found out that the young man was a very skilled carpenter but had recently lost his job. He told my friend he had found some side jobs but had to turn down some lucrative cabinetry jobs because he didn't have all of the necessary tools...the very tools that my buddy no longer wanted.

Without hesitation, my friend told the couple about his flirtation with woodworking and the tools he had recently stashed away. He asked if the young man would like to take the tools off his hands, at no cost other than the gas needed to drive his truck over to the house. The young man almost fell to the ground. He could barely get out the word "yes" before the cashier threw her arms around my buddy and tearfully thanked him.

My friend had the best time bringing the young man to his house and helping him load up his truck. Please keep in mind these weren't a few hammers and nails but some fairly pricey pieces of equipment. My buddy told me that he saw the young man choke up a few times, and all he could say was, "This is a miracle...how can I ever thank you enough?" In the end, my friend and his wife became friends with the young couple. Today, that young man does very well for himself and his family. My friend recently converted his shed into a "man cave." He has a foosball and pool table in there and a very nice, elaborately built bar...handcrafted by a very grateful young carpenter with some cool new tools. What goes around comes around!

Gather up all the stuff that's in perfectly good condition but just sits around your house unused. Trust me, there is someone out there who needs it. You will make more room for yourself and help another person at the same time.

The act of giving is one of the most satisfying things you can do. When you are feeling a little disconnected from your passion, you will be surprised at what giving does for you. It opens you up to others. It allows you to access a part of your spirit that you may not always be aware of. It gives you the chance to be a light for another person. When you give, the truth is, you receive. You receive good feelings, happiness, joy, and blessings. As your gift leaves your hand to be received by another, in that moment, from inside of you, you will know passion and inspiration. It will become tangible, and you will want more. Give, give, give. Then give some more.

CHAPTER

7

WHAT IF? WHY NOT?
(BEING MORE FEARLESS)

If you step on your fears, you climb a lot higher.

We all know about fear. Some have said it stands for **F**alse **E**vidence **A**ppearing **R**eal. Some describe it as paralyzing. Some say it is something that "crops up." Regardless of how you categorize it or describe it, we have all experienced it in one way or another. Sometimes it is irrational; sometimes it is factual. Some of us are afraid of dying. Some are afraid of dogs. Some are afraid of creepy crawlers like spiders, bugs, and snakes. Some are afraid of bullies. Others, heights. And still others, public speaking.

We all may define fear differently, yet we know it when it shows itself. Often what we are afraid of most are the challenges that life presents to us. Situations that seem just too scary for us to handle on our own. Conversations that we are worried about having. A confrontation you know you'll have to have the next day and that keeps you up all night because you're dreading having it.

I believe there is a "secret" to dealing with challenges. I don't believe that it is the challenge itself that brings on fear, but often that is where we focus 100 percent of our attention. Instead, I would suggest, as have many wiser people before me, that it is how we react to the challenge that is so much more powerful.

The fear-inducing challenge may be the present place you find yourself, but where you are standing does not mean as much as where you are going. It is what we do in that moment, between feeling afraid and taking action, that makes all the difference in the world.

For example, you may find yourself anxious and fearful about talking to someone at work about something they did that had a negative impact on you. Perhaps they said something disrespectful in a public forum so you stay up at night worrying about it. You rehash their words, how they made you feel, who was there to overhear, over and over again. All of the negative emotions start to bubble up and they literally make you feel bad. Your stomach hurts. Your head aches. You can't sleep.

Your fear has taken you over. Of course, the reality is that you won't be able to serve yourself, your loved ones, or your colleagues well when you are fearful, anxious, and sleepless.

WHAT IF? WHY NOT?

What if instead of focusing on the circumstance, you focused on a fear-fighting to-do list? If you are lying in bed, sick to death about something, it is better for you to get out of bed, make yourself some decaf tea, grab a pen and paper, and devise a plan. Have a strategy. Come up with a plan of attack. (And no, I don't mean a plan to jump the person who was mean to you in the parking lot! Don't get carried away!)

One of the best ways around the paralysis of fear is to take action. Start to live by the "What if? Why not?" mantra. Einstein said, "Nothing happens until something moves." So true. Want to get into shape? You have to move off of the sofa and into the gym. Want to become a leader in your organization? You have to move towards studying the job description, practicing your interview skills, and updating your résumé.

So with Einstein's quote in mind, I want to give you a new way to think about your FEARS: **F**inally **E**nergizing **A R**eal Solution. When you stop worrying about the what-ifs, you can finally take action toward a more successful life, inside and outside work. When you put your energy into taking the action needed for a solution, you leave little energy to feed into the excuses and paralysis that fear seems to bring into your experience.

So let's energize a real solution! Grab a pen or sit at your laptop. Make a list of the things you are afraid of or that are making you anxious. So if, for example, someone had said something disrespectful to you in front of others and you were afraid to confront her about it, perhaps your list would look like this:

1. I am worried that if I confront her she will say something even meaner.
2. I am worried that it will escalate into a big fight.
3. I am overwhelmed by her sometimes. I find it hard to debate her, and it stresses me out.
4. I am scared she will retaliate since she often makes the schedule.
5. I just am not very good at confrontation.

Now, try "What if? Why not?"

So you might write, "What if...instead of worrying about what she may or may not say, I take ownership of the fact that I am not a doormat and I am a mature, articulate person? I can certainly get her alone, where there is no audience for her to play to, and let her know that she hurt me. If she chooses to speak unkindly, I can point this out to her and ask her to rethink what she is saying. I don't have to allow her words to affect me. I can let her know that just because she thinks I am a _____ doesn't mean I am. What if I let her know that her disrespect goes against not only normal social behavior but is also a violation of our work standards? What if I decided to act and speak in this way? Why not?"

All you have to do is take your fears and then imagine "What if" you did or said something, i.e., took action in some way, that maybe in this exact moment you're afraid to do. And then after you write that all out simply add "Why not?"

As simplistic as this exercise is, it is amazing how empowered it will make you feel. "What if? Why not?" allows you to take that fearful thing and attack it with voracious action. Your focus is no longer on the circumstance(s) causing your fear but rather on the best possible strategy for addressing it. Taking massive action in any given situation has an amazing effect. You start to see yourself as a more powerful individual.

EVERYBODY FAILS—IT'S TRYING AGAIN THAT MATTERS

Do you know what is often the difference between a very successful person in a given work environment and a very unsuccessful person?

Usually, it is simply action. Successful people don't sit around all day saying, "Well, I could do this...but...." They get off of their "buts" (pun intended) and start doing.

The most successful among us weren't usually handed anything. They rarely stumbled into success. Instead, they had to create it. They took action. They didn't wait to be told to do something. And you know what? Along the way, they failed. Surprise! They didn't take action and succeed every time, and that's okay.

It always makes me chuckle when a person in public life, like an actress or an athlete, is referred to as an "overnight sensation." While overnight success is certainly possible, it is extremely rare. Usually, those who've been deemed "overnight successes" have actually been studying, practicing, auditioning, working out, training, receiving coaching, and falling flat for years. It's their passion, their willingness to get up one more time, to take one more action that led to their success.

Think about the biographies of some of your favorite artists. Most successful bands were turned down and kicked out of dozens of record company offices until they finally signed a deal and went on to win awards and sell massive amounts of records.

It is hard to believe, but the foundation of success is often failure. The hard, sharp, ugly rocks piled beneath the smooth and symmetrically poured foundation are what really hold up the castle. Those "rocks" anchor the structure. No, they aren't pretty, but they serve a purpose.

Also, remember that success and failure are really not final destination points. They aren't "islands" in the ocean where you land and stay forever. Success and failure are more like the waves in the ocean. They come and they go. No one is successful at everything that they do, nor is anyone always a failure. Sometimes the waves are huge and lift you high. Sometimes they pull you under. Sometimes the waves are small and tickle at your feet. Regardless, understand that success and failure's waves aren't there to break you; they are there to teach you.

"What if? Why not?" starts with the premise of possibility—what if? It allows you to go beyond the mere circumstance you find yourself in and instead start to focus on a cure.

Imagine if medicine or healthcare was 100 percent about diagnosis? That's it. You would go into the ER and the doctor would say, "Yes, we figured out your problem. You are having a heart attack. Good luck with that. No need to thank us; that is what we do. So see you later." Well, that's no fun! All they did was tell you about your circumstance. What you need is some action. Actually, your very life depends on action, and that certainly goes for your work life.

Just like a heart attack would require action and treatment in order for you to survive, your willingness to take action addressing that which makes you fearful requires action as well. It is the same thing. You must Finally Energize A Real Solution.

GET *REAL*

"What if? Why not?" also ends with the premise of...possibility. It is asking yourself, *Why would I not do this?* It allows you to not only diagnose what you are afraid of but to have that "real" conversation with yourself. That conversation leads to a realization that what you are afraid of is not as powerful as what you can do about it. (*Please*, read that last sentence again!)

You cannot be passionate if you are afraid. Passion and fear each require immense energy, and you simply cannot feed both states at the same time without causing great psychic harm to yourself. You cannot get results if you are fearful. While you might certainly be able to lash out or react fearfully, you won't see the same positive impact had you instead applied possibility and action to the fear.

Is it fluffy to be fearless? No. It's actually quite brave.

What if you put down this book right now and began to create a plan to address a "fear," thereby energizing a real solution?

Why not?

CHAPTER

8

WHAT'S REALLY IMPORTANT?

A life spent on the small things leads to a small life.

This past Christmas I was absorbed with the usual stuff we who celebrate Christmas are usually absorbed with. I was planning the menu with my wife for the dinner we were hosting. I was making sure that we bought all the Christmas gifts for the kids. I was getting ready for the pre-Christmas cruise we were taking with our friends and our kids.

The tree went up the day after Thanksgiving, and we decorated every nook and cranny of the house with a decoration or two (or five). In pursuit of the goal of having my house and yard to be visible from the International Space Station, I went back and forth to the store what felt like 25 times to buy just one more strand of lights or yet another light-up decoration for the front yard. It was the fun type of chaos you both enjoy and grumble about. The last thing I had on my mind was cancer.

WAKE-UP CALL

Just before Christmas, my wife, Dawn, was diagnosed with cancer. She has the most positive attitude and brightest spirit, along with a great sense of humor. When we got the call that the biopsy confirmed cancer, I remember we were lying there quietly and she chuckled. She turned to me and said, "When I was making my Christmas list, I don't recall putting cancer anywhere on it...."

What followed was a mix of good news and bad news. Bad news—surgery and radiation. Good news—a very treatable type of cancer with an almost guaranteed cure ahead. Bad news—her feeling so tired she could barely lift her head and needing to be away from our two-year-old for ten days following radiation. Good news—follow-up exams were excellent and she managed to look beautiful and keep smiling through it all.

It was certainly a life lesson. I can see how it affected her for the better. She just doesn't let silly things get to her anymore. She seems a bit calmer. She's not worried about as much. She actually told me that she was *grateful* for the whole experience because it scared her into realizing "what was REALLY important." It has had the same profound effect on me.

I recall going with her for one of her appointments at the Cancer Center. I was not in a good space. I was bummed out. I felt sorry for her, our kids, and embarrassingly, myself. I was quiet. She noticed it since...well... I'm never quiet.

We were sitting in the waiting room and I felt a mix of anger, resentment, and sadness. *Why her? Would she die? How is our toddler going to handle this? Will she need to be away for long?* All sorts of thoughts like that. I was so absorbed in my own pity party that I didn't even notice anyone else sitting around us.

Then, I heard laughter, and it caused me to look up. A couple, not much older than us, was sitting across the room from us laughing at something they had seen on the TV in the waiting room. She was in his arms and leaning her head on his shoulder. She was wearing a kerchief on her head to cover her baldness caused by the chemo. She was very thin and her skin looked gray. Her eyes were sunken. I noticed the I.V. port inserted in her chest and the bag of fluid infusing. She was quite obviously very ill. In fact, my observation of her physical appearance based on my 20 years in healthcare was that she was very likely terminally ill.

Seeing her in his arms, I hoped I was wrong. I abruptly excused myself from the pity party where I was the only attendee and came back to reality. I started to look around the waiting area. At least from what I could tell, Dawn was probably the healthiest person amongst the patients there at that moment. I realized that while her situation was no picnic, it paled in comparison to what was around us.

I put my arm around her and kissed her. I told her I loved her. I excused myself to go outside, saying I wanted to make sure I had locked the car but really it was to have a good cry. I needed to cry. I cried because I felt bad for the patients in that waiting room and all they and their loved ones were going through. I lost my dad to cancer when I was 23, and I know personally how much it hurts. I cried because cancer absolutely stinks. I cried because I was grateful that I was realizing what really mattered.

For that couple across from us, what really mattered was that they had that moment, that embrace, and that laugh. How many more did they have? Heck, how many more do any of us have? I'm willing to bet that their list of what matters had changed over the last several months. Why did it take a life-threatening diagnosis to remind me of what was really important? I don't know. But that's what it took.

At that moment the laughter from someone who some might say probably has less to laugh about than we do smacked me on the head and woke me up. I walked back in that waiting room feeling a little different from when I had left it.

SEEING THE BIG PICTURE

When things happen at work or anywhere in life that set you off, ask yourself, *Does this really matter?* You may absolutely come unglued or become deeply hurt when some family member "unfriends" you because they don't agree with your politics or don't like the team you're rooting for. While it feels bad, does it really matter in the big picture? Is it going to ruin your day? What if this is your last day on this earth? What if this is someone you love's last day on this earth? What if this is the unfriending offender's last day on this earth? Kind of puts it into perspective, doesn't it?

So much of the stuff that we worry about, at work and elsewhere, is not what really matters. Not only that, but usually the things we are worried about don't even come to be. It might be what we talk about; it may be what we worry about; it may be what we spend time losing sleep over... but does it matter? Usually, no.

What *really* matters to you? Finish these thoughts:

1. If I had six months to live, I would want to_____.
2. If I could never see or talk to_____ again, I would want them to know_____.
3. If I could do one positive thing at work or in my profession/field, it would be to_____.
4. I would love to spend more time with_____.
5. I would love to spend more time doing_____.
6. I would love to know/learn more about_____.
7. With all of my heart, I love _____.

These are just to get you going. Spend some time on these. Like, maybe stop reading and do it *right now*. No...really, I'll wait.

Did you answer them? (I hope you didn't write in the actual spaces, because that makes it a lot harder for you to resell the book when you're done!)

When we think about being more passionate about our work, we have to be very clear about the obstacles in both our thoughts and actions. One of the biggest is letting insignificant things slow us down. We will so often focus on the issue du jour or the person making the most noise rather than the stuff that truly matters. If you could have back every minute of your life you have spent worrying about utter nonsense, you would probably add a few months if not years back to your life.

Often we make the mistake of focusing on the trivial things in life and blurring that which is most important. We need to be aware of this and allow ourselves to wipe clean our lenses and refocus. *When we make the mistake of focusing on that which shrinks us, we cannot expand; we cannot grow. When you don't expand or grow, you experience inertia. When you experience inertia...eventually, you cease to matter at best and cease to exist at worst.*

At the end of the day, the things that really matter are the things you would die for. The things that really matter are the things that if taken away would be crushing. Take some time to sort out what *really* matters. When you know that, it truly sheds some light on the things that really *don't* matter. This is an exercise that makes a difference. Do it. It really matters.

CHAPTER
9

OVERWHELMED OR "THERE'S SO MUCH ON MY PLATE, IT'S SPILLING ONTO THE TABLE!"

Think of the things you make time for...are they worth your time?

Alright. So, how can I write a book about engagement and the obstacles that impede it without addressing feeling overwhelmed? Honestly, I can't, so here it goes. Perhaps you're thinking, or have thought, *I'd love to try forgiveness...but I'm too busy!*; *I want to take some time to come up with a plan for dealing with psychic vampires...but I'm too busy!*; *It would be awesome to make some time to gather together some books and clothes to donate but... wait for it ...I'm too busy!*

Okay, I think you get what I'm saying. Sometimes it feels like we are just too busy to do the "fluffy stuff." If you feel that way, own it. There is no shame in this game. If you feel that you are "too busy," you just might be. Nothing applies to everyone, so I know there are exceptions at certain points of our lives. But I promised you at the beginning of this book that I would make you uncomfortable and I'm about to do that now. Here it is: You're not too busy to do this stuff.

Oh, you are mad at me now! Now please understand, since words mean things, I didn't say, "You're not busy." I said, "You're not too busy to do this stuff." There's a huge difference. Yes, you are busy. Most of you are not hanging around work or your home even saying, "Gosh. There's nothing to do! I wish there was something to do..." Life is busy. Don't get me wrong. *You* are busy. So am I. But I'm going to argue that we are NOT "too busy" to take care of ourselves.

BUSTING THE "TOO BUSY" MYTH

Here's my case...Your Honor(s), may I approach the bench?

First, you've got to be real about your time.

(Now here's the caveat. There are *periods* in our lives, maybe long periods, where things are unusually crazy. I have a friend who is finishing their PhD, selling their home, changing jobs, and going through the process of adopting a child. I know, right? This is on top of working full time, taking care of the house, and balancing their relationship. Busy. Busy. Busy. But this is not the "norm" for them. So, yes, there are times when "too busy" fits. But even that will pass.)

What do you spend your time doing? You need to decide how this best works for you when you analyze it, but you will probably find it easier to start with categories like this:

1. Work (meetings, assignments, breaks, meals)
2. Home/Chores (cleaning, laundry, repairs)

3. Self-Care (e.g., showering, sleeping, eating, gym)
4. Commuting/Traveling
5. Leisure/Down Time (TV, going out)
6. Family Commitments (kids' activities, caring for parents, pets)
7. Appointments (hair, doctor, dentist)

Generally, this may cover most, if not all of the categories that fill our lives. If you think of more, or if you have different things that fit your life, add those as needed. Once you have established your categories, put each one on a different page of a pad or notebook. (You are taking notes, aren't you?)

Next list all the things that fill your day and approximately how much time they take. For example:

Wednesday:
Self-care: Shower: 6:00 a.m. – 6:20 a.m.
      Dressing: 6:20 a.m. – 6:42 a.m.
      Breakfast: 6:42 a.m. – 7:00 a.m.
Commuting: 7:05 a.m. – 7:35 a.m.
Work: Emails: 7:40 a.m. – 8:00 a.m.
      Meeting: 8:00 a.m. – 9:00 a.m.
      Staff meeting: 9:00 a.m. – 10:00 a.m.

And so on. Don't worry about jotting all of this down as it happens. It's perfectly fine to do it after the fact. Just do it as soon as possible so that you don't forget how long each task took.

Choose to do this for at least one weekend day and three weekdays—so maybe Wednesday through Saturday. This will give you a great idea of where your time is going. You need to know this so that you can determine where your time is spent. Think of this as doing a "time budget." If this is too complicated for you, or if you're not a detail person, simplify it. Just like with a financial budget—knowing how you are spending your money to determine how best to save it—doing this with your time gives you the same outcome.

I mapped out how I was spending my time, and I was quite surprised by the results. For example, I travel quite a bit. On travel days, I found that I was rushed leaving the house. Therefore, I had the impression that I was "just too busy." In reality, I was just trying to cram too much— finishing up my packing, grabbing a bite to eat, preparing what I would wear on the trip, etc.—into a short period of time. When I saw how much I was trying to do on those travel days, I was able to figure out a better plan.

I now look at my travel week the night before. I pack everything I can so that the next morning I do not have that on my list. All I had to do was rearrange my after-dinner ritual slightly to free up some time that I then used to pack. I found that simply cutting out one short TV show, or recording it so I could watch it in bed when I was relaxing later, and paying a neighborhood kid a few bucks to give the dog his evening walk gave me the time I needed to complete key tasks the night before traveling so my travel days weren't so hectic.

The result? On travel days, I had a little more time to spend with my kids before I left, run a last-minute errand, or finish another important task. I made small changes, but the effect they had on lowering my stress was anything but. Instead of rushing around wondering "where the time had gone," I could now sit on the floor and race cars with my three-year-old. By the way, he always wins! Aren't toddlers little characters?

So, one way to make a small dent in your "I'm too busy" life is to really figure out where your time is going. You may find ways to make simple adjustments. For example, maybe leaving your house 10 minutes earlier actually saves you 30 minutes of traffic! Maybe you are able to budget a few dollars to have a hardworking teenager cut the grass on Saturday, or you can sit the family down and delegate a few chores to take some of them off of your plate.

My point is, we get so used to saying, "I'll take care of it..." that change seems impossible. Maybe cooking that big pot of pasta sauce on Sunday can also cover dinner for two other nights, saving you time. Maybe instead of going to the store three times a week, you could make a list for the whole week and go only once. Maybe you can buy your movie tickets online and print them at home, saving you 15 minutes of waiting in line. Perhaps you can schedule short morning "huddles" with your staff or coworkers so that information is shared, problems are looked at, and issues are addressed, so that you actually save yourself time during the day putting out fires.

Where are you really spending your time? Once you know that, determine where you can adjust to allow for time to do things that improve your life. Make this your mantra: "I will spend time getting better rather than spend time getting by." Get a little obsessive about this. It's worth the time.

Now that you've scraped a few morsels off of your full plate, make some commitments to yourself. First, commit to playing more offense than defense in your work and life. While there will always be crises to deal with, unless you're a Navy Seal, this should not be the entirety of your work.

PLAY MORE "O"

Now, of course, I'm being somewhat facetious in that many of us have jobs like Navy Seals where crisis is the actual job. When I was an ICU and then a Trauma nurse, my job had a lot of crisis built into it. I'm not talking about the crises that come with your actual job description. I'm talking about the issues and problems that you are constantly having to address and that suck the life out of your day so that you are always playing defense (reacting) rather than offense (preemptive strikes).

What does playing more offense look like in practice? Well, if you're a leader and you spend a lot of time dealing with employees who come to you with complaints, you should stop waiting for them to come to you (defense). An "open door policy" is fine, but it isn't okay to use that as your primary way to communicate with your team. (It's also a bad way to manage a relationship! "Hey, honey, anytime you want me to tell you that I love you, just come to me and ask me to tell you." Yeah. See you in family court!)

Go to your employees. Frequently. Round on them. Ask them specific questions about things that you know they care about based on your past conversations with them. If they always seem to be asking you about getting more supplies, maybe you could round on everyone monthly and ask, "Do you have enough supplies to effectively do your job?" Then, if they say, "No," you get that stuff for them. Getting those supplies for them before they run out helps you avoid a time-consuming crisis and the added stress that comes with it. It is always easier to put out a few smoldering leaves than to extinguish a forest fire.

Listen to your employees and proactively seek out the very things that you can do to make their lives better. The benefit as it relates to managing your plate is that by playing more offense you will have more time to do things that you love about your work. And doing more of what you love will fuel your passion. Seek every possible way to play offense.

You don't have to be a manager for this strategy to work for you. For example, if you're in healthcare in a direct patient-care role, you can round on your patients to determine what they need. You can play offense by meeting those needs on your terms and according to your schedule so that you are not constantly being pulled all over the place.

If you do any kind of service work where you have customers or clients, the same strategy applies. Ask them, "What is one thing I can do for you today to best meet your needs?" Move away from, "If you need anything, let me know..." When you do that you're giving your time away. Instead, be proactive.

Some of you may be in sales and do regular sales calls. In fact, they're probably part of the job. Perhaps you also do calls where you are just checking in. Here is where you can look for ways to proactively serve. Customers can sense a sales call a mile away. Don't be offended, but sometimes they will avoid it. However, if they start to grow accustomed to you sending an email or calling to make sure all is going well, to ensure they are satisfied with the product, and to ask if there is anything that you can do for them, I promise, the sales will roll in. They will appreciate the "servant attitude." Not only that, but you will limit the "emergency" calls you get when there is a disaster.

For example, if you happen to check in with someone and they mention that the screen on the XCWV3000 that you sold them keeps flickering (I just made that up, so if you actually have such a thing as an XCWV3000, I hope I didn't just jinx you.), that's actually a good thing.

You can upload new software or get tech on it now rather than later when it turns into a 2:00 a.m. freakout call from your customer because the system rebooted and will now take six hours to get back online! It's easier to deal with a flicker than a shutdown! Play offense rather than defense in your work. It is a surefire way to save time and to limit those panic-button-pushing moments that cause your adrenaline to shoot through the roof.

LIGHTENING YOUR RESPONSIBILITY HOARD

Often we get overwhelmed because we have allowed ourselves to lose control. We get swallowed up and covered up by "stuff." Have you ever watched that show on television about the people who hoard things? It's almost always the same sub-plot. Something happened in their life, and they took in one item and then another and another and so on, until one day they're so overwhelmed with stuff that their house is being condemned.

Obviously, the deep emotional and psychological issues they're suffering from make it much more complicated than that, but there is an important similarity between how they let their life be taken over by literal stuff and how the rest of us let our lives be taken over by all of our responsibilities at work and at home. You may not be hoarding plastic knives, old magazines, and cans of peaches, but you *are* hoarding issues, problems, and complaints. And those can be even more "condemning" than the most militant housing inspector.

You get bogged down by the hoard of responsibilities in your life when you use "Let me know if you need me..." as your primary way to get information or to problem solve. That's playing defense. It put you in a position where you have to be mostly reactive. Then all of a sudden you are getting bombarded by, well, people letting you know that they need you. Why? Because you've given them that power.

Had you played more offense and reached out to them periodically to address their issues, you could have done so on your own time rather than having to do so when you are already in the middle of 17 other things. Or at the very least, it may have been a somewhat more manageable issue that you could've gotten on top of before it blew up into a big disaster.

Here's another way to look at it: I would much rather the airplane mechanic responsible for maintaining the planes I regularly have to fly on be proactive and ensure everything works well before the plane takes off. I hope he/she played offense and took the time to look for problems. I would really hope he/she doesn't play defense and think, *Well, if the plane goes down, I will do everything I can to learn from it and make sure it doesn't happen again.* Oh, heck no. Make sense?

Life and work will probably not get "easier" for most of us anytime soon. Let's not hope for easier. Let's hope that we can make the effort to get better. Look for the areas in your life where you can take back a little of the power. Be proactive. Play offense. Clean off that full plate and get it in the dishwasher.

CHAPTER

10

TAKING ACTION

No traction without action!

I mentioned earlier that Einstein said, "Nothing happens until something moves." I'm including it again here because I think it is a beautifully simplistic way of observing life. What a simple truth. You won't get a paycheck unless you move off the sofa and go to work. You won't get into shape until you move off the recliner and into the gym. You won't finish that degree until you move your eyes off the TV and into your books! Simple but true.

I read somewhere that the primary reason people don't accomplish their goals or get things done is...they don't even try. What? No way! Yes way. No complicated research is needed to find the cause. Simple neglect is the answer. The absence of action results in the absence of results. Period.

So what to do? As Einstein would say, and I paraphrase, "Move!" Usually the best way to begin to accomplish something is to take immediate action. Think of something at work that is getting in the way of your being what you desire, whether it's being more purpose-driven or more inspired. Now, think of something that you're putting off.

For example, maybe you feel that you'd be better off professionally if you achieved a certain certification/degree/title, etc. But you're struggling with all of the "stuff" that clutters your mind and gets in the way of getting it done. For many of us, this is so normal we don't even know anything different. Do you ever notice that you obsess over details but not in the most meaningful way?

FIGHTING ANALYSIS PARALYSIS

Maybe your process goes a little something like this: Let's say you want to paint a picture. But instead of obsessing over the image in your mind that you just have to get onto the canvas, you focus on where you should buy the paint. *Will you have time to do it before Tuesday? What if they're out of the paint you want? They probably are. They almost always are on backorder. That stinks. Now you'll have to go to that other place across town to get the paint. You hate that other store. It always smells like cheese in there. The parking is a nightmare. Last time you went there someone dented your car. Speaking of that, when are you getting that dent fixed? You probably should do that instead of painting. How can you be creative with a dented up car? Now, where did you put that card with the body shop information on it...*

If this is at all similar to your brain process, welcome to my world! Sometimes we really want to accomplish something, whether it is a painting or a PhD and we just can't seem to get off the ground. It can be ADD (that is actually my personal diagnosis, although I don't think they called it ADD when I was a kid—they just called it "detention") or just a simple failure to take action.

Maybe the infamous "analysis paralysis" is the cause. You fail to launch because you can't get out of the "research and development" phase. You start to spin so many details inside of your head that it becomes almost impossible to move. You are paralyzed because all you can do is analyze different aspects of the situation. One thought leads to another and still another until you're not even thinking about your goal anymore. Instead, you've ended up, as in the painting example, wondering when to get your car fixed.

I want to share something with you that is so deceptive in its simplicity that you will think I am being dismissive of this issue. I want to assure you that I am not. As Van Halen would tell you...go ahead and jump! Just do something. Anything that is an action leading towards the goal. It can be something small or something major. Nothing creates action like action. It is truly a domino effect.

BECOME AN ACTION HERO

If you have been spending the last seven months "thinking" about getting that certification, you could probably admit that is more than enough time to think about almost anything. As soon as possible, log onto the website and order the book you need to study. Maybe even spring for the extra three dollars to expedite the shipping! Already have the book? Great, you already did something. Commit to reading for 15-30 minutes each night when you get into bed. If you don't want to miss the *Housewives of Butter Lake, Minnesota* (it is inevitable they will get a show, I am sure!), record the show and watch it later. It's so much better to be able to fast-forward past the commercials anyway.

The idea here is this: If you *think* about something, that's great. If you can manage to take *action* towards achieving it, that's a lot better.

Commit to being an "action hero." Look at the things in your life that you wish to accomplish. Certainly this can apply to work or your personal life. Then list three to five things that you can do within the next 24 hours to advance toward achieving that goal. Then list three to five things that you can do within the next week, month, three months, and six months. Create this list with check boxes so that you can check them off. If you're tech-savvy, create a document or grid for this and upload it onto your online calendar.

Please don't let the simplicity of this throw you. The great majority of people in this world don't write down their goals. Honestly, if you did 10 minutes of research, you would probably find that the great majority of people don't even have goals! It is simple to do things. Yes, I know there are often deeper reasons why people don't, but getting too deep into that just postpones accomplishing your goals even more! So, just do something. Anything!

Seven months of twisting a thought through your head and thinking about all the reasons why you could or couldn't do something will not get you as far as 15 minutes of action. Sure, you may discover the "thing" isn't what you truly want. Good! Now you can figure out something better. You may find it will take longer, be more expensive, be more involved, or be more difficult than you previously thought. Great! Now you can plan accordingly. Most likely you will find that you've simply put off doing something that is not that difficult and once accomplished can add good things to your life.

Years ago I wanted to fulfill my goal of working in a Trauma Unit. I had been pretty comfortable in my role as a Pediatric ICU nurse and I wasn't sure if I could swing the new learning. My friend took the dive before me and was really enjoying the change. He would visit me weekly on his break and almost beg me to transfer. I remember telling him, "I would, but it is a three-month internship!" He looked at me and said, "Three months are going to go by whether you do it or not."

Ain't that the truth? I could spend three months learning something amazing or spend three months thinking about how it would take three months to learn something amazing! So, I jumped. Three months flew by, and I had some of the best experiences of my career working with smart, amazing, inspiring people.

Order that book. Sign up for that seminar. Reach out to that person. Put on those workout clothes. Make that doctor's appointment. Do one thing, today if possible, to advance you towards that opportunity.

Be an "action hero." But maybe without the headband, robot sidekick, and explosions all around you, unless you really need that to get you fired up!

CHAPTER
11

KINDNESS

Kindness is a language that everyone understands, but unfortunately, not everyone takes the time to speak.

I strongly believe there are way more kind people out there than unkind people. Oh sure, the meanies make themselves known loud and clear on the roadways, in store lines, and in schoolyards. And yes, there have always been and will always be mean people. Storytelling as far back as Greek mythology, Shakespeare, and the Bible (remember David and Goliath?) have featured monsters and meanies who want to ruin your day.

The M.O. of these monsters is to scream the loudest, make the most noise, and take up the most room. In other words, they want to make their presence known and to intimidate the kind people around them. Usually those who are gentler, kinder, and more concerned with helping others rather than stomping through Tokyo, crushing buildings and shooting fire rays from their mouths, go through life in a less demonstrative manner. That said, because the meanies in our lives are so good at making their presence known, sometimes it seems like they're everywhere. But trust me. Kind people are everywhere. They're the majority.

Many of us have been fed the propaganda that "nice people finish last." Sure, sometimes that is exactly what happens. But it is certainly not the hard and fast truth that we're made to believe it is.

Gandhi spoke about being the change you wish to see in the world. I will never tire of rolling that mantra around in my mind. I want it to be so deep in my soul that it becomes my norm. (And if you haven't figured it out yet, this is going to be the fluffiest chapter yet! Embrace the fluffiness!)

There is no better way to change your world than through kindness. I hope you've already noticed the elements of that kindness message that I've woven throughout the book. When I first began writing it, I wanted that message to be almost subliminal, but, taking my own advice, I am jumping into this headfirst. If you want to have a better work life, a better personal experience, try to find a way to be purposefully more kind.

KINDNESS FOR A CHANGE

Today's workplaces, not to mention everything else in our lives, seem to be in a constant state of change. The economy, our savings, the value of our homes, the cost of living—it has all undergone significant change compared to just a few years ago.

Our approach to our work has changed as well. It's different. Organizations, leaders, managers, and all of us frontline employees are looking at our work in ways we never did before. First, many of us either know someone who has, or personally might have, taken having a job for granted. There was a time when many of us assumed we would never have trouble finding or keeping a job. Now, of course, we know better.

There was a time when many organizations, certainly those in my field of healthcare, assumed that their biggest problem in the future would be simply recruiting more people and finding the room to expand their facilities and services. Now, many of them are struggling to survive and are looking at cutbacks and layoffs. Some of the organizations that are around as I am writing this book won't be by the time it hits the shelves. That's simply where we are.

Many of us are looking at everything differently than we did before. Everything. We are not only looking at how we balance our budgets and pay our bills; we are looking at how we relate to our work. Is it enough to simply do what we have to do? When things get tough, people take stock. When times get challenging, it is often our nature to begin to do a little inventory. Where before, our "work" was more focused on growth and advancement, for many it is now becoming more obvious that this is not enough. When I talk to leaders and frontline folks, I hear much more about engagement. It's almost as if the "fluffy stuff" is being looked at with more of a serious eye.

Part of the engagement process involves how we "feel." It is hard to feel "engaged" when you feel a sense of animosity or anger rising out of the organization where you work. While there are many great ways to deal with the psychology of this, I believe there is a faster, more direct way to change the "feel" of an organization. It is an often overlooked, misunderstood, and underestimated thing. It's called kindness. Ring any bells?

THE KINDNESS CURE

Being kind. Receiving kindness. That probably sounds like an overly simple cure, but often it is the simple things that make the biggest difference, isn't it? Think about it. Sometimes relationships can be healed when someone simply says, "I'm sorry," or, "I love you." Sometimes a child's banged knee needs only a small kiss from mommy or daddy, which despite not containing antiseptic or anesthetic relieves the pain. Sometimes a plant simply needs...watering.

When I've had an organization share with me that they struggle with engagement and I've asked, "What have you done so far to address this?" I have NEVER, not once, had any of them say, "Well, we looked at ways to increase the level of kindness in the organization." So, doubt if you will, but if you haven't tried it, how can you say it won't work?

Do you feel that kindness is a part of your working environment? Is it directly expressed in the mission or vision of your organization, or is it at the very least implied? Is it in your goals to be kinder? I think, at least for the majority of us, the answer is "no."

So how does kindness fit in to engagement?

Let's start by addressing what many of you are probably thinking right now. *No*, I don't live on "Inspiration Mountain." *Yes*, I do know that this world of ours really isn't all that kind most of the time.

How often in your daily commute do you see a person go out of their way to move up behind the car in front of them rather than let someone cut over? How often do you see someone jump in front in a line when it is clearly not their turn? How often do you hear someone make snide, rude, judgmental, and flat-out unkind comments about others, often first saying, "I don't mean this in a mean way..." or, "I don't mean to gossip..."? (By the way, I've found that the best way to know someone means something in a mean way or is about to gossip is if they first say they are NOT doing that...just saying.) Yet, there are great lessons in kindness even in these acts. Khalil Gibran once said, "I have learned silence from the talkative, toleration from the intolerant, and *kindness* from the *unkind*; yet, strange, I am ungrateful to those teachers."

In other words, we certainly owe a debt of gratitude to those who have shown us great examples and lessons in kindness—our family members, the Gospels or other religious lessons, our teachers, and other mentors. But we shouldn't overlook that there is much to learn from those who, well, have it all wrong.

Imagine how your life would change if every time you observed or even were the recipient of unkindness, you simply depersonalized it and had an attitude of gratefulness for what you've just learned. It is one of the greatest things that you can learn to do.

Why am I starting from this perspective? Because we are all good at making excuses and too often we go into victim thinking. "Oh, the world is a tough place; no one is kind anymore. It will just eat you up and spit you out...I will just be kind to those I love and hold close and the rest are fair game...." Good luck with that. It's too easy to be a child and simply say, "No one else is doing it. Why should I?" When you were a child, it was okay to think and act like one, but we need more people embracing their grown-up-ness and moving to a more enlightened place.

So, yes, there are mean, unkind people in the world. Quite a few actually. There are people who look out only for themselves. There are bullies. There are people who don't care who they hurt or step on. And people who believe that if you're nice or kind then you're weak.

Maybe you have picked up on the fact that while some of these people do get some of the goodies the world offers—the most candy dropped from the piñata, more money because of their dishonest dealings, a really attractive and/or wonderful mate—they are almost always *some of the most miserable, depressed, and disgusting human beings you've ever met!* Yes, unkind people do often reap the rewards of this world. But no matter what, those rewards are certainly temporary and don't necessarily mean they're overwhelmingly happy.

Even the pharaohs learned that all of the worldly power and influence they could muster, being treated like gods on earth and striking fear in everyone around them, mattered little in the end. Sure, they filled their crypts in the great pyramids with astounding treasures, but where did that treasure go? With them? No. It gathered dust. It was just stuff in the end.

So it is childish to look at some unkind person who cut to the front of the line to get the biggest piece of cake as "winning" anything. After all, we know how that story ends. Do you know any really happy, engaged, self-actualized, spiritually fulfilled people who are unkind? No. You do not. So, to say that the best strategy for your life is to join them should seem to you, when you meditate on it, absolutely foolish.

That's why I wanted to start with this aspect of kindness. It requires reflection and a change in thoughts. It requires you to make the decision to stop saying, "No one else is kind, so why should I be?" You're bigger than that. Instead of emulating the bad aspects of the world, learn from them and move to a better way.

In the quote from Gibran, I believe the wisdom in what he is saying is simply that we are fortunate to not only have people show us by great examples how *to be*, we are actually just as fortunate to have people show us how *not to be*. I am just as grateful when someone gives me great directions to get somewhere as I am when someone includes in those directions what streets or areas to avoid as there are dangers lurking. By telling me where not to go, they are saving me some pain. The wisest amongst us pay attention to those directions. To ignore them puts you in jeopardy. So, steer away from "Unkind Street." The only thing that lives there is more suffering for this world of ours.

LET'S TALK ENGAGEMENT!

So, now that all of *that* is out of the way, it's time to make the engagement-kindness connection. For employees to be engaged, there needs to be an atmosphere of kindness. People have to feel it around them. It is hard to stay engaged or become engaged in an environment that lacks kindness. It is not impossible, but it is definitely harder. One of the best things organizations can do—and let's be clear, an "organization" is not the walls and the landscaping; it is the people—is to begin to talk about and focus on kindness.

How? Start by thinking about how you recognize kindness. You know it's hot outside or raining or cold by what you see, hear, and feel. Recognizing when kindness is present isn't much different. Ask yourself:

1. What does kindness look like? How would I see it or visualize it in my workplace?

2. What does kindness sound like? What words or phrases can we say at work that radiate kindness?

3. What would make me feel that someone was being kind? Is it an action that they take? A favor that they do? Words of support or encouragement? A smile? When do I feel like I am receiving kindness, and could that be something that others may be able to relate to?

It is also helpful to consider the opposite side of these questions. In other words, what does it look, sound, or feel like when people are being unkind at work? What is it that someone can do or not do that makes me feel as if they are not being kind? This all goes along with the Gibran quote I shared earlier in the chapter.

When someone speaks sharply, doesn't look you in the eye, doesn't greet you, smirks while you are talking, interrupts, or uses disrespectful tones or body language, you can probably recognize those all as unkind behaviors.

Understanding what "kindness" looks like and what "unkindness" looks like is like getting directions that tell you what streets to turn onto and what areas to avoid. Asking these questions about kindness and unkindness is a great project to do on your own and as part of a team. Often just asking and answering the questions above are enough to not only get the ball rolling on bringing kindness into your workplace, but to also score a goal with the ball!

Start there.

Then move on to doing some of the work of creating kindness. First know that it starts with you. Hopefully, there is a whole group of "yous" who want to bring kindness into your workplace, but even if there aren't, you have to take the initiative to infuse your organization with kindness.

How do you "find the kind" inside of you? Well, even if you're Oscar the Grouch, your inner Elmo is not far away. (Sorry, I have a three-year-old. I haven't watched grown-up TV in my house in awhile!) Here are some suggestions:

1. *Send thank-you notes.* Buy a box of thank-you notes and spend some time on a day off, a flight, a train ride, or whenever you have a free second filling each of them out, expressing thanks to anyone you think deserves it. This could be a coworker, teacher, manager, waiter, running buddy, dog trainer, babysitter, etc. Just go through the whole box and fill them out. I mention this method more than once in the book because it is an easy way to accomplish so many great things!

    We are losing the blessing of thank-you notes in our society. In times past, these and other forms of written correspondence were precious things. I bet your grandparents probably have a box or two of written correspondence they've kept. The written word has a permanence, a tangibility, that even spoken words lack. Letters and thank-you notes are there to go back to over and over again.

    For those of us who love to read, there are probably books we've read more than once. As a youngster, I read *The Cross and the Switchblade*, *The Outsiders*, *The Hobbit*, and other favorites dozens of times. I knew the stories by heart, but it was the reliving of the moments that expanded my mind or gave wings to my spirit that brought me back. For people of faith, there is a reason they read and reread their religious books and lessons. They find comfort in the stories, in the words of peace and wisdom.

Thank-you notes do much of the same thing. They are often a written expression of kindness that offer reassurance, support, and yes, even love to the recipient. And after you give them out, trust me, people will reread them over and over again. To play on a quote from Quint Studer, don't underestimate the difference a thank-you note makes.

2. *Go back to the chapter on "Giving."* Read it again, and if you haven't yet taken action then please go for it.

3. *Pay it forward.* If you live in an area that has toll roads, keep a few extra coins in your car (if you can afford to do so), and commit to paying the toll of one person behind you once a week or once a month.

4. *Look for ways to be kind.* When you walk into your place of work, quietly ask yourself (or your higher self, or God, or your invisible friend Hugo) to show you someone to be kind to. I will promise you one thing. Someone will appear. I don't know if it is all that mystical of an event, although it could be.

    For me personally, this is more of a spiritual experience, but either way, I think it does come down to focus. You are focusing your thoughts on finding someone to be kind to. Your subconscious is now on alert. It's like you're casting a net, and even though you may forget the net is there, it catches someone in it. That someone may need to laugh, cry, hug, or $3.55 for a latte. Just ask and you shall receive. And so will they.

Okay, these were just a few of the simplest examples. Of course, there are many more ways to be kind. Kindness can be shown through acts of charity or by sending positive thoughts or prayers. Kindness can be sent via email or in person. Kindness can be the "look at me!" type or the "don't let your right hand know what your left hand is doing" type. Of course, you may define kindness differently from me. But let's not fight over the best type of kindness. Just pick what works for you and go for it.

If you want to prove me right (Why would you want to prove me wrong? That's not so kind!), do a quick Internet search on keywords like "kindness + improving immunity," "kindness + health," "kindness + happiness," or anything similar. You will find, as did I, what many of us already suspect: Kindness is...good. Yes. Good for you. Good for me. Good for our health and our mental well-being. In fact, value-wise, kindness probably outperforms the stock market and the price of gold.

All kidding aside, one of the greatest ways to stay connected to passion, to stay engaged, to lock onto success, and to find an inner sense of happiness is to incorporate kindness into our work. Can you clean up a mess that isn't yours? Can you carry something for someone? Can you make sure to compliment someone on their suggestion in a meeting, their font on their PowerPoint presentation, or their amazing cleaning technique? If you do this, with purpose and intent, every day, you will not only feel better about your day, you might make others feel better about their day.

Who knows, your acts of kindness may act similarly to that stone in David's slingshot. You might knock a monster right off of a skyscraper in Tokyo. How cool is that?

CHAPTER

12

GOING IT ALONE

We can carry more, do more, achieve more, be more, and go farther...as a team.

For many of us, being seen as "tough" at work is essential. I work in healthcare, and I can tell you we have some of the toughest people in the world in our places of work. I mean, you have to be pretty tough to deal with what we deal with. We see blood, death, violence, pain, screaming, crying...and that's just in the Finance Department! But seriously, this leads all of us to become somewhat tough.

When you're thought of as tough, you feel like you have to be able to handle everything yourself. Isn't that the truth? I mean, a tough person doesn't ask for help! Can you imagine? We are tough people in our workplaces. We are like warriors! Vikings! Pioneers! Oh wait, that's good, pioneers. Let's stick with that.

Think about pioneers. Almost every country or culture has had their version of pioneers. I am from the U.S. so I'm going to use our pioneers as my example as I am most familiar with them. So think about the pioneers who settled the American West. They didn't need anyone. They went it alone. Didn't they? They had no maps. They had no street signs. They just packed up their wagons and went at it.

On the surface, it sounds so impressive, doesn't it? That "go-it-alone pioneering spirit"! But think for a moment about the reality of what they did. While we hold pioneers in high esteem for their bravery and guts, there is another, darker side to their stories. It wasn't all that safe to be a pioneer. That go-it-alone attitude didn't always give great results.

OH, PIONEERS!

When we think about pioneers, we picture a world where they all built their own personal "little house on the prairie." But for every pioneer who made it that far there were ten who got eaten by bears! Don't laugh. There was a lot of bear-on-pioneer violence back then. It's true. Going it alone can be a bear!

And it can be just as risky to go it alone at work. Okay, maybe not eaten-by-a-bear-level risky, but risky nonetheless! It is simply common sense that we are much more effective when we work together. We can carry more, learn more, fix more, repair more, heal more, and understand more when we work as a team. But even though we intellectually grasp this concept, most of us still struggle with doing it.

While we supposedly higher-functioning beings still struggle with working in teams, the animal kingdom totally gets it. Picture, if you will, the plains of Africa. Imagine a herd of wildebeests galloping across the savannah. Off to the side, a lion, or a tiger maybe, is stalking the herd.

Now think back for a second to all of those animal shows you've watched where a lion is stalking a herd of prey. Be honest. Which wildebeest always seems to get the claws and the fangs? Which wildebeest is always the one that becomes the main course for the lion? Is it ever the wildebeest running in tight formation at the center of the herd? No. Never. It is never the wildebeest working well with the other wildebeests.

Which one gets chomped? You know the one! Everyone knows a wildebeest like this...the wildebeest that always gets eaten is the one that has wandered away from the herd. The one that got distracted by a flamingo taking flight or saw something shiny in the trees and went it alone. Which wildebeest gets it? I will tell you—the wandering, distracted, pioneering wildebeest!

There is great danger when we go it alone. Yet we make the decision to do so almost every day at work, and frankly, also in life. How often have you had a coworker or a friend outside of the workplace make a decision or take an action that blew up on them? Afterwards you probably thought, *If only they would've asked for help!*

While many of us have been conditioned to believe that we look "weak" when we ask for help, we have to understand that often we truly ARE weak when we are slammed to the ground and broken by the "pioneering" actions we took instead of asking for guidance or advice. I'm sure you'd prefer "looking" weak to "being" weak. So, great, I have you somewhat convinced that it would stink to be a wildebeest (actually, they do look kind of stinky, just saying). So, what to do?

Funny you should ask; I have some suggestions:

1. *Take advantage of coaches.* The greatest athletes in the world
    all have a coach. So do the greatest teams in the world. Every
    Super Bowl team or World Cup Soccer Champion team has
    a coach, actually several to be honest. My employer, Studer
    Group, calls the folks we deploy to work with our partners
    "coaches" and for a good reason. A coach is in the game with
    you. They have skin in the game.

    As a matter of fact, when a team has a bad season, it is
    most often the coach who gets the blame (or fired) as a
    result. Think about the last basketball or football game you
    watched. What was happening on the sidelines? If I had to
    guess, I'd say the coach of the losing team was probably losing
    his mind at some point, certainly more so than the players on
    the team. The players were probably looking bummed, but
    the coach looked like his head was about to explode! Why?
    Because the coach sees the whole picture and wants that win
    as much as or even more than the team sometimes.

    A great coach often leads to a great team. (Look at the amaz-
    ing results Studer Group's partners get if you need convinc-
    ing!) So, you need a coach. Find someone who knows your
    job/field/profession very well and who has gotten great
    results. This could literally be someone you work with on a
    regular basis whom you simply admire because of their out-
    comes or work habits.

    Ask them to "coach" you. Have them observe you doing your
    job for a period of time and then ask them to offer you their

impressions or critiques. You will be amazed at how helpful this could be. If you are in sales, have someone who is great at it watch you with a customer and then offer you advice on what you did well or could do better. If you teach, start IVs, repair stuff, or collect payments, have someone coach you. Seeing your work through another person's eyes may open yours!

2. *Learn more.* Go to seminars, classes, or institutes and be around others who are interested in what you do. In healthcare, we are fortunate as there are literally hundreds of these. Studer Group has the very best ones for healthcare. (See some resources at the end of this book!) When you are around others who do what you do and you participate in these events, you will be surprised at how much you learn even by osmosis! You will talk to people, share war stories, listen to speakers and teachers. There is no reason to go it alone. Go to a seminar, take a class, surround yourself with other like-minded wildebeests!

3. *Bring a speaker to your organization.* Sometimes it is actually more cost effective to bring someone in to speak to your team than to bring your whole team to a conference. When you do this you really get major benefits. I speak for a living, and it is always amazing to me to be able to spend time with a team and watch them grow before my eyes! A speaker brings his or her knowledge and understanding right to you and a good one brings the team together. Take advantage of great speakers/presenters. (And whaddaya know, there are some resources for this at the end of the book!) Look me up! I'll be there!

4. *Make a friend at work.* It has often been said that to have a friend you need to first be one. Amen to that. Reach out to peers at work and try to establish some afterwork get-togethers. These team-building events can have very positive results. I know of a few organizations where individual departments take it to the next level and rather than just go out for food or whatever, they get together to do community service like building houses for the poor, working at soup kitchens, or visiting folks in retirement homes. What a cool idea! Clearly they realize that not only should we not go it alone, but we should know that there are others who are alone who could use a little lift up.

We are just not meant to go it alone. As I look back over my years in healthcare, I think of the many people I took care of who were dying and had no one. No family. No loved ones. I remember elderly people brought in from nursing homes like forgotten discarded coats. Children, left to die, abandoned like toys on a playground, by parents who were in prison or on the streets. Human beings. Our brothers and sisters, our children and babies, left to take a last journey alone.

WORKING TOGETHER FEELS BETTER

But in my more than 20 years of work in healthcare, I rarely if ever saw that happen. No, it was a nurse, or a physician, or a firefighter/EMT, or a police officer, or an environmental worker, or PT, or RT, or unit secretary who would hold that lonely hand as a last breath was taken. That task was never assigned. Never once. No one begins their shift and needs to be told, "Go in there and hold that child's hand as she dies...." We just did it. Why? Because we knew to. It is inside of us. I believe it is inside all of us. For some it is part of our daily work; for some it is not. But I think it is a human thing.

We understand deep within our spirit that no one should die alone. It is simply wrong. We are not meant to go it alone. Going it alone may at times sound "brave" but truly there are inherent risks. Too often we become burnt out because we simply refuse to own the fact that being a pioneer can lead to more problems than it is worth. It is exhausting to load the wagon, feed the oxen, and build that log cabin alone. While going it alone may lead to discovering the occasional gold mine or establishing a home on the range, you also run the risk of being eaten by lions and tigers and bears...oh my.

CHAPTER
13

SPEED BUMPS

Challenges can be speed bumps or deep potholes: A speed bump tells you to slow down, get rid of what's rattling around, and tighten up what's squeaking...a pothole breaks your wheels, traps you in place, and ends your progress.

When my wife, Dawn, was diagnosed with cancer, everything seemed to feel different. I felt like I was seeing life through a foggy lens. For those of you who have experienced this personally or had a loved one go through this, I'm sure you know exactly what I mean. If you haven't, I can describe it to you. It feels like when you have the flu but you still go through the motions of life. You're dragging, foggy, and everything feels like it takes twice as long. Fun things seem less fun, and normal things feel like torture.

I found myself going into "nurse mode." I'm sure all of you nurses out there know what I mean. For those of you in other professions, "nurse mode" is probably not all that unlike "cop mode," "executive mode," "firefighter mode," "parent mode," and "physician mode." It's when you put yourself and your feelings aside because you need to fix something, accomplish something, or save someone.

And I was experiencing it to its fullest extent. I decided I was going to fix her cancer by being super-husband and super-dad. I would do every possible chore, clean the house until it squeaked, be ridiculously positive, spiritual, and inspiring, and have our two-year-old doing algebra and quoting Shakespeare. Easy, huh?

In life, as in work, we often have challenges, and sometimes these challenges throw us. In life it can be illness, break-ups, divorce, and the like. At work it can be layoffs, conflicts, poor staffing, an overloaded schedule, and leadership changes. These are like speed bumps in many ways. I learned this from meeting Aretha Franklin in a grocery store. Okay, not really her, but someone who reminded me of her.

SUPER-DAD'S KRYPTONITE: YOGURT

When Dawn had to have radiation, she had to be away from our then-two-year-old and me for ten days. Our wonderful friends Jason and Tyler, who lived 300 miles away, moved her into their house for this time and surrounded her with love and warmth. We have awesome friends!

I decided I was going to be super-dad. Luke, our toddler, and I would be holding down the fort. I had this, I reassured myself. I could do this. All was going to be well! No sweat!

I found myself keeping busy, really busy. Like organizing-the-junk-drawer-daily busy. Then Tuesday came and I had some groceries to buy. Luke was at school for a few hours so I headed off to the store. Tuesday mornings are a great day to grocery shop. The place was empty. I had a list organized by aisle, grocery type, and section to expedite the process. (I know, right?) I was organized and prepared. When I grocery shop, I am like a Navy Seal.

I made my way to the dairy section. Milk, eggs, and Luke's yogurt were on my list. As I filled the cart, I found myself reaching for some lemon-flavored Greek yogurt. This was Dawn's favorite. A staple in our fridge. As I picked it up, I realized I was deviating from my list. After all, Dawn would be gone for another nine days. Why would I need to stock up on her yogurt?

Then the weirdest thing happened. As I stood there holding the yogurt, "Dawn's yogurt," I had a thought. It was a like a train horn in the distance breaking through the gloomy silence of my mind. I thought, *What if Dawn gets worse?* Then, staring at the yogurt that I didn't need to buy, I thought, *What if the cancer spreads?* That train was getting closer. *Could she die?* The train tracks were shaking. Then I wondered, *Is this what it feels like when someone you love dies? You hear songs, go places, or pick up yogurt that reminds you of them and you realize that you'll never see them again on this earth?*

The train pulled into the station. Then it happened. Everything that I had been avoiding thinking about, pushing back, keeping busy in order to hide from poured out. The yellow yogurt container blurred before my eyes. I felt steam pouring out of that train engine, but it wasn't steam dampening my face, it was tears. Real, salty tears pouring from my eyes. I began to cry right there in the dairy aisle.

THE WISDOM BOMB

Now, let me be vivid. I am not talking about a subtle misting of the eyes. No, I am talking full-on grown man sobbing. Big time. Clean up on aisle six! My baby blues have sprung a leak! This may have gone on for a moment or two before I became aware of a presence just to my right. As I looked up from my tear-soaked yogurt container, I realized there was a woman standing in front of me. She had a look of deep concern on her face. Her right hand was up as if she wanted to reach out to me but wasn't sure if she should. I can only describe her as beautiful. Glowing. She looked remarkably like Aretha Franklin. The glow from the frozen vegetable cases behind her illuminated her like an angel. She was a vision. *I* was a sight.

My sobbing subsided slightly and I looked up. I normally would've been embarrassed but emotion had taken over. She worked up the courage to touch my left arm. In a strong but gentle voice she asked, "Baby, are you okay?" I couldn't yet speak even though I wanted to. I didn't want Aretha to think I was a lunatic. All I could muster was to lift up the yogurt container as if this would offer an explanation.

She looked puzzled. Gripping my arm she said, "Sugar, yogurt should never make you cry!" We both paused. A shift took place. Then the train changed tracks and a cloud lifted. We both burst into laughter and were like little kids giggling. I've often thought that if there was a security camera recording this event, it must have been hysterical. It was exactly what I needed. Release. Laughter. It broke down a wall. A wall I didn't even realize I had built.

I told her everything about the cancer, the radiation, and why the yogurt made me cry. This total stranger. A kind face. A gentle human being. An angel really. An angel I've named Aretha listened to my whole story. All the stuff I was holding in poured out.

LIFE GETS BUMPY

After my outpouring, Aretha looked at me, *into* me, really. Then, she dropped a "wisdom bomb" on me. She said, "Honey, sometimes God throws speed bumps onto your road. But these aren't meant to break you. They're meant to take you to another place. That's what a road does, honey. It's a means of travel. It's a path. Think about a speed bump, now. What is it there to do?"

I thought for a second and I said, "Slow you down?"

Aretha's eyes lit up over her glasses and she said, "Exactly! Challenges, like speed bumps, are there to tell you to slow down. You've been running on full speed, trying to fix things, and you haven't yet slowed down and digested all that you're dealing with. So speed bumps tell you to slow down and pay attention to the road. Look at the trees. Be careful you don't run over anything that can cause you delays on your path."

She paused and smiled. "Let me ask you what else you might notice about a speed bump. When you ride over it, you might hear some stuff clacking around in your trunk. Some tools you forgot back there, beach chairs from a trip to the beach way back when, and other stuff. That speed bump reminds you that you might be carrying around some 'stuff' that you need to be rid of. Maybe that stuff needs to be put where it belongs. Maybe it needs to be thrown out."

She continued, "The other thing you notice when you ride over a bump is sometimes you hear rattles and squeaks coming from that chassis.

When you ride over those bumps, they let you know there might be some things that need to be tightened because you've allowed them to become loose. Sometimes, you might need to add some oil to something because the road you've been on has caused some rusting to take place. That's wear and tear from the journey."

She paused so I could take this in. She straightened her spine and looked me dead in the eyes. "Honey, this bump is telling you to slow down. Get rid of the nonsense that is rattling around, distracting you and weighing you down. Tighten up and oil up the stuff that has gotten too loose or rusty. Let me ask you, is your wife's prognosis good or bad?"

I answered, simply, "Good."

"Okay," she said. "Take that on the road. Are your kids okay? Do you have a job? Can you make ends meet? Are you healthy?"

I answered, "Yes, ma'am...."

"Good. That's what you put in that trunk. Those what-ifs that got you crying aren't speed bumps; they're potholes. And if you linger there too long, they become sinkholes and they will swallow you up alive. You drive over a speed bump, honey, and you keep going. You learn and you move on to the next one. You got me?"

I weakly answered, "Yes."

But that wasn't good enough for Aretha. She was demanding some r-e-s-p-e-c-t! Sharply, she asked, "I said, *you got me*?" Her tone woke me from my trance.

"Yes!" I exclaimed.

We both laughed. We talked for another minute or two and I thanked her for her kindness. I told her she was a blessing to me that day and that it felt like she appeared like an angel. Aretha laughed and said, "That's a first for me. I been called a lot of things, but an angel? That's a new one!" She gave me a big motherly hug and looked at me wordlessly saying, "You're gonna be alright." And for the first time in many days, I believed it.

Then my angel named Aretha turned on her heels and disappeared behind the frozen food aisle. What an experience.

That day, Aretha told me exactly what I needed to learn, what I needed to hear. Isn't it amazing that when the student is ready, sometimes an angel appears?

When we have challenges, at work or in life, we have choices. We can treat them like potholes and we flatten our tires, bang our heads on the roof, skid around the road, and maybe even get stuck in place, spinning our wheels, making that hole deeper and deeper. Or we can treat challenges like speed bumps. We can slow down. Dump what isn't helpful for the journey. Tighten up what has become loose and oil that which has become rusty.

Challenges aren't meant to break you. They're meant to take you farther down the road, slower, lighter, and smoother.

CHAPTER
14

BURNOUT IS A GOOD THING! (WHAT?)

When you're hungry, you must eat. When you're tired, you must rest. When you're thirsty, you must drink. When you're burnt out, you must feed your spirit.

Okay, of course, I don't really mean everything about burnout is good. But I've come to view burnout as a sign of hope. Here's why.

Ready? Here it is: *Low performers don't get burnt out!* Did I just blow your mind? Only people who care, and care deeply, about their work get burnt out. People who don't care don't get burnt out! They're not even exerting enough energy to do the minimum, so why in the world would they tire themselves out *caring*?

My point here is this: If we are seeing burnout all around us, if we ourselves are burnt out, that means we care or at some point cared deeply about what we're doing. Most people who are feeling burnout are usually higher performers! Higher performers care! The low performers aren't even in the equation. They're too busy hiding out so no one asks them to pull their weight! They're in front of a mirror somewhere mastering sarcastic eye-rolling techniques.

YOUR BURNOUT SHOWS YOU CARE

So, the silver lining of all that burnout we are seeing is that it means there is hope. You get burnt out not because you're a bad person—quite the contrary. You get burnt out because you have given so much, cared so much, offered so much, and never took the time to refill. People who are burnt out are not lost causes. Burnout is often a simple sign of compassion fatigue. It can be cured. Burnout sufferers are not the *Titanic*, sinking fast. They're a sailboat in need of some new breezes, and to get them they simply need to turn that boat around and fill that sail with wind.

You bring a lot of yourself to your work. You show up physically by using your physical strength and abilities when necessary. You show up mentally by bringing your decision making and professional judgments. You show up intellectually by calling upon your training, smarts, and education to get the job done effectively.

Most of all, though, you show up spiritually. You bring a sense of "self" to your work. If you're teaching and one of your students is struggling with the lesson because they lost a parent, are sick, or had to move out of their house because of financial issues, you feel it.

If you're taking care of the sick, and a patient gets bad news or takes a turn for the worse, you feel it. If you're leading a sales team, a finance team, or a work crew, and the company is announcing layoffs or pay reductions, you stay up at night worrying about how it's going to affect the lives of those you work with. These are more than "feelings." For most of you, these workday difficulties engage your spirit. You bring a lot of yourself to your work. You can't be engaged if you are disengaged from your spirit!

Think of a bottle of water. It starts out full, but every day you pour out a small amount. After awhile, if you're pouring water out of the bottle but you never add anything back to it, what happens? Right! Eventually, it will be empty! An empty bottle. That's burnout. You, the water bottle, were once full, but because of the overflow of giving and never replenishing, now you're empty. Burnout!

How do you refill an empty bottle? You go to the water cooler and you open up the tap. Within a moment or two, boom! You have a full bottle. Refilling the human spirit is not much different. Oh, we can complicate and over-analyze, but in truth, it is pretty straightforward.

WHO'S GOT SPIRIT?

You need to find the "source" of whatever it was that once filled up your spirit. When did you last feel like your spirit runneth over, so to speak? For those of you who need a more straightforward question, when was the last time you felt on purpose, excited, fired up, joyful about your work? There's probably a great story behind this. It could've been 22 years ago. It could've been last Wednesday, but when was it? When you figure it out, ask yourself these questions:

1. What was going on?
2. Where were you?
3. Who were you working with?
4. Why was this time or experience so fulfilling?

5. What did it feel like? What words would you use to describe your feelings at that time? Excited? Energized? Giddy? Pumped up?
6. What was being said at the time? What words do you hear when you think of this experience, if any? What was the conversation?

When you reflect back on that time, you might find that it was a day when you encountered someone who needed your help or expertise. Perhaps, you were able to take that person from a "bad" place or state to a "good" one through what you do. In other words, you did your "work," made an impact, and felt awesome.

Let me make this specific using an example.

Let's say you are a Human Resources staff member or leader. Maybe a few years back you came across an employee who was going through a tough personal time, and they came to HR to resign. They were struggling with personal issues (family stuff, kid problems, etc.), didn't feel appreciated at work, and were in the process of making arrangements to take a less demanding job. They were in a dark place, and it's possible that they were not seeing the big picture. They were just giving up. The only alternative they saw was to quit.

For whatever reason, you connected with this person. Their story got to you, touched you. These situations are what you got into HR for! Perhaps you think back on this day and you remember making a personal connection with this person.

You showed them there were alternatives to leaving the organization. You let them know how valuable they were and that you didn't want to see them throw their work away because present circumstances were rough for them. You were maybe able to brainstorm a way that they could maintain their position while working a schedule that allowed them to address their problems at home. You knew that the organization recently began to offer flex schedules to accommodate situations like theirs and you were certain you could extend this to them. Maybe it was even a program you helped put into place, and in walked the perfect candidate!

By the end of your time with them, they were smiling through tears of gratitude. You showed them another way, a better way. They hugged you. You scored a major victory. You remember leaving that day feeling like this was what you were meant to do! You probably called a few friends, or your mom, or your spouse and told the whole story to share the love! Now every time that employee sees you in the hall, maybe even all of these years later, they always smile at you. And you both know why.

This is the kind of stuff I want you to think back on. When you go back there, even in your memory, reconnect to that source. The very thing that filled you up that day is still there. That ability to make a difference. To help. To comfort. To cure. To teach. To mentor. It is still there. Those opportunities are there no matter what you do. You may be in a rut right now. You may feel every day just merges into the next at work. Same old, same old. I'm here to tell you that the great thing about an empty plastic water bottle is it can be used over and over. Even when it starts to fall apart, guess what? It can still be recycled!

So, the "source" for replenishing your spirit can be found by remembering the time when it was most full. As you're thinking back, you'll probably remember more than one occasion when your spirit was lifted by your work. You'll start to see patterns. Maybe you find your source comes from times when you were able to be creative. Maybe you find your source comes from times when you were able to teach, mentor, or train another person.

Your source is your own. You find it, not unlike the way you would find buried treasure. There is a "map," and the map is located within the stories of the times you felt most fulfilled. You use those stories to lead you back to the source of what fills you.

See, there's some magic to this but not real magic. This magic is more like a card trick. With a card trick, it seems like the magician made the card disappear, but really the truth is much more simple. He actually just distracted you and dropped it into his pocket. Simple. Real.

The source of what fills up your spirit isn't found on some magical dimension in Wonderland. You don't have to climb onto your purple unicorn wearing your invisibility cloak while battling dragons on your way to the rainbow to wrestle the pot of gold away from a leprechaun. While that sounds like a great children's book, it just isn't real. Plus, if you told people at work that's what you were doing, HR would probably ask you to pee in a cup.

Just go back to "that moment." Look at it through different eyes. Learn from it. Create new moments that allow you to get back to doing whatever that was. Those spirit-filling moments from your past are meant to shine like a star, directing you back to your source. That's how you can fight burnout, renew your spirit, and get back to doing work that you love.

CHAPTER

15

SORRY, PRINCESS...IT'S STILL A FROG

Don't try to "kiss the frogs" in your life. Wish them well.
Be open to setting a good example. Even be a friend if it
works out that way, but stick to your own lily pad.

Not too long ago, my youngest son, Luke, was playing with my wife and me. It was a wonderful lazy Sunday. We had already run around the park and had a picnic and were now lying down on our blanket in a partially shady spot. It's a lot of work tiring out a three-year-old, but we were almost there!

Luke was sitting between Dawn and me being his usual funny self. He turned to my wife and, taking her face in his little hands, he said, "Mommy, you're my princess!" (I know, right? He's got this thing down!) In all truth, Dawn is truly a beautiful princess, so he was spot on. Of course, this brought a huge smile to her face. Luke then turned to me and said, "I didn't forget you, Daddy. You're a prince!" (Man, he's good!) This resulted in a group hug all around.

But Luke is never one to go halfway. He grabbed both our hands and he said to Dawn, "Mommy, kiss your prince!" Lucky for me, she did. Dawn and I giggled but then looking towards our son, we both noticed he had all of a sudden become extraordinarily serious. He was staring at me as if I were a strange alien that just jumped out of a cloud or something. Finally the silence broke when he leaned towards me and as serious as can be said, "Daddy, are you going to turn back into a frog?" Good to know he had been paying attention all of those nights when we read him fairytale bedtime stories. Leave it to my son to be able to reverse engineer the whole "kiss a frog and turn him into a prince" bit. But it got me thinking.

EXERCISE IN FUTILITY

How often do we think that we can change a person? Sometimes, especially at work, we spend inordinate amounts of time trying to change someone. Sometimes we even convince ourselves that it is for "their own good." But that gets tricky, doesn't it? More often than not what we find is that while it is great to want to set a good example or to mentor someone, to hope to change someone is often an exercise in futility.

Often our burnout comes from putting our energy into the wrong things. If you drive a car in the opposite direction of where you need to go, eventually you not only run out of gas, you're even farther from your destination. When you spend your time trying to change people around you, it is the same thing.

If I had a dollar for every time someone has come up to me at a conference where I've spoken and said, "Rich, I'm a pretty inspired person. I could be even more inspired, but there's this one person I work with who just drives me nuts. Can you give me some coaching on how to fix them?" I would be quite wealthy. (Actually, with today's economy, I may have to adjust that dollar per comment up to a dollar seventy-five. Just saying.)

I pretty much always have the same answer. I usually say something like, "Well, I probably can't suggest anything to help *that person* but I do know one person who can make that whole situation 100 percent better...." Then when that person says, "Really? Who is that?"...I point at them and say, "You."

You can kiss all the frogs you want, but the only things you'll get in return are weird looks from the other people picnicking by the pond or kicked out of the park by the park ranger for animal endangerment. And maybe a few warts too!

This idea that work would be better if other people acted better is maybe somewhat true, but it is mostly beyond your power to create. I say mostly because you may be in leadership and have the ability to counsel people or dictate how they should or shouldn't act, but I'm not talking about that. And even if I were, sometimes the people who suck the joy out of you aren't violating a policy or a standard. I'm talking about those of us who work side by side with a peer and we let their words, deeds, attitudes, behavior, mood swings, or what have you change us. We then lament to everyone that if only for this person things would be perfect.

Stop trying to kiss that frog.

WHAT MAKES YOUR FROGS SO FROGGY?

Usually these people are triggering something within you. There's something that they do or say that brings up something inside of you that causes you to feel as you do.

It's funny, when I've talked to groups of people and also had one-on-one time with the same group about this topic, I've found that one princess's frog was another one's prince! Sometimes that "irritating" person doesn't affect another person the same way they affect you. (Many of us might even be shocked to find out that someone thinks we're the frog!)

When you think about the person who you've given so much power to that they have the ability to give or take away your passion, ask yourself why it is that what they do impacts you so much. I mean, unless they are verbally or physically abusing or assaulting you, what is it? Why are you letting them get to you?

The only person who should have power over your level of passion or inspiration is you. For real.

The list of ways that people "get to us" is too long for me to include it here, but I am going to try to touch upon the one factor that has been mentioned to me the most.

When people share with me what it is that these "frogs" do to knock them off their happy place on the lily pad, I hear things like, "She ruins my day. I can't feel good when she's around.... She's just so unhappy." Really? What a surprise. A person who makes life uncomfortable for others is *unhappy*? No! Say it isn't so!

Of course they are! Happy people don't make you unhappy! (Okay, unless you're an unhappy person already and then, yes, happy people might make you unhappier.)

So, basically what you're complaining about is that you want to be "happy," but there's an "unhappy" person around you—so then you can't be happy? So that means you can be happy only if everyone around you is happy?

That's going to be frustrating.

Here is a great question to ask yourself in this scenario: *What does their unhappiness have to do with me?* Why in the world are you owning their unhappiness? If they're very gassy, are you going to own that too? (Now, to be fair, working with a very gassy person might be a real challenge to staying engaged!) The truth is, you don't own, control, or have responsibility for that person's unhappiness.

Your work is not to make them happy. Your work is what your calling in life has brought you to do within your field or profession, and you should be doing it with passion and heart. So if you're taking on that person's unhappiness, stop it. No, I mean it. Stop it! You can do that, you know? Their "unhappiness" is just a thing. It's like a hat or a shoe or a cup or a pencil. It can't do anything to you unless you let it. Walk away from their unhappiness. Don't give it time. Don't give it words. Don't give it energy. Don't give it one tiny bit of power.

Keep in mind that I'm not saying you don't have to engage with the person, talk to them, or work with them. That probably isn't your choice. But you don't have to engage with, talk with, or work with their unhappiness. When they are complaining about how horrible the day is, staring off sullenly into space, rolling their eyes, or sighing like a lost moose (Do moose sigh?), and you feel that lump in your stomach coming up, let it go. Open your heart and speak quietly to that feeling, as that's all it is, and laugh at it and say, "Go! I don't want you here!"

It's like performing a frog exorcism. Be gone from me, evil frog! This is easier than you may think. Feelings are things. Just like you can toss away a gum wrapper, you can toss away a feeling. You have to be honest and acknowledge it for a moment (like you would an old gum wrapper by feeling it in your hand), you have to hold it briefly (like a gum wrapper), and then, like when discarding a gum wrapper, you make *the purposeful and conscious choice to pull back your arm, aim it towards the trash bin, and release the gum wrapper!* Do you then worry about the gum wrapper? Do you go back into the trash and pull it out so that you can carry it around all day? No, you don't. You toss it. It's gone. It's not yours anymore.

TAKE BACK THE POWER

I know this might be somewhat esoteric for some folks, but I would be failing you if I didn't talk about this next topic. I'm not trying to sound like a yogi or anything. The only yogis I know are Bear and Berra. I've got nothing against either of them. But this is something that bears your investigation. As human beings, we often give power to things that we shouldn't. Giving power to someone else to dictate our level of joy is crazy.

Let. It. Go.

That feeling that comes up for you is coming from somewhere. Maybe when they talk or act in a certain way that demonstrates their unhappiness, it reminds you of someone or something in your past. Maybe it was how that kid in third grade who bullied you used to act or speak. Maybe it was a parent or an ex. It's not like you need to be Sigmund Freud to realize that sometimes our "triggers" come from things that have happened to us in the past.

But seriously, folks, take the power away from it. If you can figure out what this person's actions or words do to you, distract yourself. Do something else. Don't give it space in your head. Think of something that you love as soon as you start getting that lump in your belly. Picture your dog or your boat or your child. Something! Change the trigger. That way you're working on changing the only person you have the power to change. Yes. I am pointing to you.

I want you to own that when you say that another person at work is not "allowing you" to feel as inspired as you can that is simply an excuse. You are avoiding the truth. That truth is this: It's not what they are saying or doing; it's how you're thinking about it. Let me be as direct as I can be: *Don't you ever give another human being that much control over who you are, how you feel, or what you do. Ever.*

These feelings are not things you have to carry around. You don't have to think about them. The feelings that are coming up for you are things that you can simply let go. Is it easy? Probably not. Neither was learning how to walk and talk but you got that. It's actually something that you have to work at, constantly. But to achieve freedom, you will have to break a sweat. It is what it is. It gets easier as you practice it. Take that first step. Speak that first word of freedom. You won't know what you can do, until you do.

Even as you try this and progress, you will still have that moment where you "feel" the pain, but rather than it sticking with you all day, week, pay period, or year, you acknowledge it. You feel it. Like that gum wrapper, you aim it and you make the choice to toss it away.

So don't try to "kiss the frogs" in your life. Wish them well. Be open to setting a good example. Even be a friend if it works out that way, but stick to your own lily pad.

CHAPTER
16

NOTICE THE YELLOW CARS IN YOUR LIFE

I don't want to be full of only good; there's no such thing as "good-ful"...I want to be full of great; I'd rather be grateful!

Have you ever heard an unusual name? One you've never heard before? Over the course of my years in healthcare, I have heard some names that were unique to say the least. Doesn't it almost always seem that after you hear the unusual name the first time, all of a sudden you start hearing it everywhere? You hear it on a TV show, read it in a book, see someone interviewed on the news with the name. Seems to be all over the place!

Why is that? I think the science of the mind explains that well. I have often heard it said that what we put before the mind, what we focus on or give attention to, causes the mind to be more aware of that thing.

So for example, you meet someone named Pluto and all of a sudden you see a TV show about Pluto on the science channel. (I don't think I will ever get over the demotion of Pluto from a planet!) Your kid comes home from school with a Pluto the dog sticker he got for being well behaved. Your friend on Facebook posts a picture of their new puppy named...you guessed it! Pluto! Seems to be everywhere. It may be that because you entered the name Pluto into your awareness now your brain is extra sensitive to it. You see it everywhere now, because you first saw it in your brain.

I ask this next question in front of some fairly large audiences, the largest being almost 2,000 people. Here it is: Do you drive a yellow car? It is rare that I get even one or two people to raise their hands, even in a large group. Okay. My bet is, while there may be a few of you reading this who do have a yellow car, most do not. So here it is:

Yellow car. Yellow car. Yellow car. Yellow car.

Guess what's going to happen? Today, after you put this book down (hopefully you're not reading and driving) and begin your drive to work or home or wherever, you're going to start seeing yellow cars everywhere! I mean it.

You're going to think I went to your town and rented yellow cars and had my posse drive them all over town just to prove myself right! I promise you I didn't. I don't really even have a posse. Those yellow cars were always in your town. That neighbor always had that yellow car. People didn't all of a sudden go out and get their car painted yellow. They were always there. You just had no need, or call, to notice them. But now that I called your attention to it, you will begin to see them. Constantly.

Becoming more aware of yellow cars won't change your life. But becoming more aware of what you are grateful for *will* change your life. Of this I am very sure.

EINSTEIN DOESN'T WANT YOU TO BE INSANE

Gratitude. People have been writing about it since the ancient days. Every great thinker, every great spiritual path, speaks about gratitude. It is a powerful thing. Luckily, it works the same as the whole yellow car thing. When you start talking about it, looking for it, becoming aware of it, purposely, you see it everywhere.

I talked about gratitude in my first book, *Inspired Nurse*. I love talking about it. I know the impact and value of gratitude on the human experience. I know and have seen, firsthand, that it changes lives.

If we agree that when we hear an unusual name or hear someone talk about yellow cars these things start popping up in our awareness, then you'd have to agree it could work the same with gratitude. So, how do you do this? Here's what I'd advocate you do:

1. *Try the 21-day gratitude game.* Here's how it works. Get a notebook or pad that you can carry around work all day. For 21 days, each day your goal is to write down one thing that you feel grateful for by the end of that day. Just one. If you have seven or ten or thirty, that's great, but shoot for at least one. You have to do this for only 21 days, and then you never need to do it again if you don't want to. Just commit to trying it for 21 days. You can do it!

    There are no rules to this. It can be anything. Maybe that day you got to work with one of your favorite people and the day flew by. Maybe your loved one surprised you with some flowers at work (No. They're not up to something. You're just *that* loveable!) Maybe it was baked potato bar day in the cafeteria, you got a good parking spot, or you won the office raffle for this book (yeah!), who knows?

Now for some, this may be more of a challenge than for others. I know. Maybe you are not one of those people who get all "fluffy" and look for the good in things. Well, let me ask you something: How has that been working for you? Have you ever heard "If you do what you've always done, then you'll get what you've always gotten"? Einstein even calls us out on this. He said that insanity is doing the same thing over and over, expecting to get a different result. More than being just a smart guy with funny hair, he also seemed to touch upon something rather spiritual. Why not be a little willing to try something different? From what I know, gratitude is not usually painful. I've never had anyone come into the ER with a traumatic gratitude injury! So, seriously, how has what you've been doing worked for you so far? If you're not as engaged as you'd like to be, then maybe the road you need to travel to get to engagement is paved with gratitude. Maybe you can even drive your yellow car on it!

Sometimes, frankly, this even comes down to fear.

People are afraid to look for what they're grateful for because they're scared they may not find anything. (You will.) They're afraid that if they start looking for what they are grateful for and start actually feeling better, then maybe something not so great is going to happen. Then, they will be more disappointed than if they would've just stuck with feeling like life stinks all the time.

That's like saying you're never going to eat at a restaurant that you love because if you taste their wonderful food then you won't ever want to eat any another food ever again. So you just eat yucky food to avoid having to experience a letdown. Does that even sound a little sane? You wouldn't want to experience good because bad might happen, so stick with bad so you can at least know what to expect.

No!!!!!

I can say with confidence that it is very unlikely that something bad can come out of your writing down what you are grateful for at work for 21 days. (I have to say "very unlikely." I can't say 100 percent because, yes, you may be walking down the hall writing down the great thing that happened, not watching where you're going and then fall down the stairs and fracture your pelvis. So I will stick with "very unlikely" just so I don't get any mean emails from anyone! So be careful out there! Don't walk and journal at the same time!) In all seriousness, you get this, right?

For most of you, the first two or three days will be weird. It might even be difficult for you to come up with something. You may even feel silly. It may feel forced. So I ask you this: Isn't it sillier to spend the day stewing about who ticked you off and what hurt your feelings? Is it better that you're maybe "forcing" yourself into feeling burnt out and stressed looking for all the bad that can happen? Either way, whether you realize it or not, you're expending energy. Use it for your betterment, or use it to stay in a rut. That's your call.

So, by day 10 or so, something starts to happen. It's that "yellow car" science of the mind thing. All of a sudden you start noticing things to be grateful for everywhere! I have met very few people who tried what I am suggesting and by the end of the 21 days were still struggling to find more than one thing to be grateful for. It's pretty amazing. These things start jumping out at you everywhere. It starts to flow. It's like riding on the yellow car highway during rush hour.

And all because you did one simple thing. You thought to yourself, *I am going to notice things to be grateful for!* Your amazing, brilliant, beautiful mind was only too happy to oblige.

2. *Play the yellow car game.* My family and I came up with this game based on my take on the whole yellow car thing. It is fun to do. You can do this by yourself or you can do this with your loved ones or friends. The rules are simple.

Every time you are driving or riding in a car, if you see a yellow car you have to call out one thing that you are grateful for in that moment. (If you're alone, it is okay to think it...although talking to and answering yourself is a lot of fun also.)

So every yellow car equals one thing you are grateful for in your life. This combines the two concepts in a fun way. Yellow cars become "triggers," if you will, for gratitude.

This is a really fun thing to do with loved ones. My family does it almost every time we get in the car. My teenager, Rhett, does it, and I've noticed as he's gotten older his gratefulness has increased and has become even deeper. Our toddler, Luke, does it, and it's pretty funny. He's probably more into it than the rest of us, just by the nature of him being so young and loving to play.

I love when Luke does this. It's fun to be driving along, thinking about whatever new thing I'm worried about that day, and from the rear car seat I hear that cute little toddler voice (Don't they sound like cartoon characters at that age?) saying, "I see a yellow pick-up truck, Daddy! I am grateful for you, Daddy!" Of course, that's my favorite! What a cool thing to cement into your child's psyche!

How many people in this world are too busy, either directly or by example, teaching their children to feel entitled and to complain? How often do you almost go into shock when you meet a child who freely says "thank you"? Isn't it sad that this shocks us? Wouldn't we all be a little better off, as a society and in the workplace, if we taught our children to look for things to be grateful for rather than to look for things to be offended by? Can I get an amen? Thank you.

Doing this creates not only a fun game to play but it creates a healthier habit than punching each other when you see a VW Bug. (Okay, we do that too sometimes! Everything in moderation, I say.) While that's a lot of fun, make sure you balance it. There's enough "punching" in our world, wouldn't you say?

This habituation of gratitude forms new pathways of thinking. You are changing your world. Well, let me be more accurate. You are actually changing the way you see your world. You are changing how you interact with your world and the role you play in it. The "world" itself, whatever that means for you, remains what it is. However, your place, your role, your energy becomes something different.

None of this necessarily completely changes the world. I mean, your becoming a more grateful person certainly will impact the "world" even if only at a micro level, but let's not overreach too much or we set ourselves up for failure. But, yes, even this small shift will have impact. There's nothing wrong with that.

PERCEPTION IS EVERYTHING

Aren't perception and thought almost everything? Isn't how you see something in your world more or less creating that world for you?

For example, let's say as a child you had a neighbor who had a huge, mean German Shepherd named Rocky. He was scary. Let's say he got out one day and chased you. He latched onto your leg and bit you hard, pinning you to the ground. You could hear him growling and you can, even today, remember what it was like to have this massive dog standing over you. The owner got to you both before Rocky could do too much damage. But of course this experience stuck with you.

So now, what do you think your perception might be of German Shepherds? You're probably still terrified of them. What they look like, how they bark, might bring you back to that day. Your "world" is not one where you want a bunch of German Shepherds frolicking.

Now shift this. Let's say as a child you weren't allowed to have a dog. But your parents had some good friends you visited regularly, and they had a beautiful, noble, sweet, playful giant German Shepherd named Rocky.

Whenever you went over to the friends' house, all you wanted to do was hug his massive neck and play with him. He followed you everywhere. You wolfed down your dinner just so you could go back outside and play catch with Rocky.

He was one of the best parts of your childhood. You loved that dog. You thought of him as yours even though he wasn't. As an adult, your inner child would come alive anytime you came across someone walking their German Shepherd. Like an eight-year-old, you'd exclaim, "Can I please pet your dog, Mister?"

Now, with that different, more positive life experience, you can easily imagine that the sight of a German Shepherd creates a whole other set of feelings. Rather than fear, when you see a German Shepherd, you feel happy and a sense of childlike wonder. German Shepherds are still German Shepherds, but depending upon your experiences with them this can lead you to some pretty strong feelings.

When you add a perception to your world, and embed it in such a way that it becomes a habit, in essence, you have changed *your* world, not *the* world. You can choose to do this for the betterment of yourself or to the detriment of yourself. Either way, you get what you ask for.

Now, let's go back to those yellow cars for a moment. What you will notice, when you begin to do this yellow car game is something pretty, well, miraculous. On the days you feel most negative, despondent, or disagreeable, it often seems like you see yellow cars everywhere.

At least, this has always seemed to be the case for me. If you pull back for a moment, you might even look at yourself and laugh. You might actually see yourself getting angry at the fact that some divine power is putting all of these *stupid yellow cars in my face!* I mean, how dare anyone get in between you and feeling miserable, right? As the kids are saying these days, LOL. If this ever happens to you, pay attention. There really is a message in there somewhere.

Each one of those yellow cars is a chance to change that day. Each one is a chance to be grateful for the fact that you can breathe, talk, sing, have someone to come home to, have a quiet house to come home to, have a job, changed your job, have a car, have a bike, have a bus pass, have eyes to see a yellow car, or someone to tell you there is a yellow car.

Each yellow car can represent a life where you win no matter what rather than a life where you are a victim no matter what. Even when life or work chases you down, bites you on the leg, and pins you to the ground, you can keep the negativity away by focusing on gratitude.

It's your choice. You can shake off negativity or choose to live a life pinned to the ground, helpless. Your choice. If you need help along the way, professional, spiritual, or otherwise, seek it and commit to doing the work. But even that starts with a choice.

The act of seeing gratitude in something mundane like a yellow car trains you to think differently. Your work life changes dramatically when you start to look for that which you can be grateful. It really, really does. Your outside-of-work life (Yes, I've heard some people have those!) changes for the better when you become a seeker of gratitude. It really, really does.

Write down what you are grateful for about your work for just 21 days. Stick to it even if it feels "fluffy."

By the way, just to lead by example, I am really very grateful that you're reading this book!

Notice the yellow cars in your life and encourage the ones you love to do the same. When you do, your world becomes something pretty amazing.

And yes, to all of my New York City friends, taxicabs can count as well!

CHAPTER
17

GUT CHECK

Sometimes you have a "knowing." Life teaches you to listen to that voice. Often you ignore it at your own peril. When you know...you know. Trust your gut.

Have you ever had a bad feeling? No reason for it. You just felt like something was wrong, amiss, askew, out of place, just not cool? You probably even felt it, literally, in your gut. Now, when you had that feeling about a person, place, or thing, did something not so great end up coming to pass? Have you noticed how that happens sometimes?

Over my years of traveling to almost every city in my beautiful home country, the U.S.A., and many in the lovely land of Canada, I have heard these kinds of stories over and over again. When I speak, I am often able to share meals or do book signings, and those often lead to my meeting wonderful people. In fact, most of this book is derived from those conversations. I literally have 10 pads of paper filled up with notes I've taken over the last few years based on those conversations.

People tell me amazing stories and share some personal and beautiful things. That's my favorite part of being a busy speaker. I learn much more from people like you than I think many of you may realize.

One thing that seems to be a steady theme is this idea of trusting your gut. I have had military nurses who were deployed in war zones tell me they had a bad feeling about going to a certain part of the base they were on and then shortly afterwards there was a mortar attack on that same spot.

I have had people tell me about having a bad feeling about renting a certain office space for their new business. After passing on that space and moving on to another, they heard that two months later there was a huge fire that destroyed the entire building.

I have met law enforcement people and EMTs who told me about having a bad feeling about a building or situation. They were thankful they "listened" to that "knowing" as it saved their lives. You're probably familiar with what I'm talking about, that sense that you "just know" something bad is going to happen. I could tell you a few dozen stories in which people I've spoken with followed that "knowing" and were extremely happy they had because it helped them avoid something bad.

THE MORE YOU "KNOW"

Do these people have some kind of magical power? No. I don't think so. None were named Merlin or Gandalf. I think this sense of "knowing" is wired into our "humanness."

Why talk about this in a book about engagement?? Because it cuts to the foundation of where this all comes from.

We know when something or someone "feels" right or maybe wrong. Look back over your life. I know there were a lot of times you might have been fooled. You may be thinking of a few exes who pulled the wool over your eyes but ended up being more like old, stinky burlap than wool!

We've all been there. It happens. But I am referring to the times when you felt something. Like a voice inside you saying, *Don't go out with them.* Or, *Stay away from that place.* I know this has happened to you at least once. I bet it may have happened in the workplace as well.

Maybe your gut told you to go for that new position and maybe you were in a "fear place" and didn't. Then someone with much less aptitude and experience got the job. And all you can do is sit back and watch that great opportunity pass you by. Or maybe the opposite happened. You felt like you shouldn't go for a position, even though everyone was pushing you to do it. On paper, it seemed perfect, but there was something inside you that said not to.

You questioned yourself, *Am I just being a coward? Is this fear talking? Is this because I don't believe in myself?* But that voice doesn't seem to be coming from that place. So, you don't go for the interview. Someone else gets the job. At first everyone just looks at you shaking their head. You start to beat yourself up about it. Then, you hear the news that the budget has been tightened and everyone in that department, including the person who got your "dream job," is being cut.

Sometimes what causes us to flail a little on the job, what causes us to get disconnected from our passion and disengaged, is simply that we don't listen to our gut. We trust everyone else more than ourselves.

Now, in my opinion, not everyone has the same level of "gut." I think like eyesight, athletic ability, math aptitude, and singing ability, your gut and my gut might be at different levels. One of us may be a little more intuitive than the other. I'm just saying this because not everyone has been given the gift of "prophecy," if you will.

I may be at a 10 on a 1-10 scale while you may be at a 3. But even taking that into consideration, I have learned that all of us have at least a modicum of "gut" instinct. I have also observed that for many of us, when we start actually using our gut, we actually move up the aptitude scale. It probably works like any other skill or muscle. Use it and improve it. Make sense to you?

So how do you do this? I think it starts rather simply.

LISTEN TO YOURSELF

To effectively listen to yourself, you have to be quiet, right? Doing so may be a struggle for most of us. I know it is for me. My brain is never quiet on its own. Never. I think if you could hear my brain, it would sound like a circus pipe organ, constantly filling the big top with that silly circus music. Constantly.

I've been told that some people call that their "monkey mind" because their thoughts are just bouncing around like a crazy monkey. Sound familiar to you? I bet some of you really relate to this. This is me most of the time. Actually, I think a lot of us in healthcare and in other high stress types of work often feel like our minds are swinging on vines from one tree to another.

Monkey mind. I love it. But I'd rather have monkey mind than sloth mind. That's just me! So this "monkey," if you will, makes it hard to be quiet, but to hear anyone you need to be quiet, right? After all, it's pretty hard to have a conversation with someone and get to a productive place when they talk over you the entire time. (Hello, Congress, take note!)

Seriously. You have to be quiet to hear another voice. And the same goes for hearing the "voice" in your head. (Notice, I didn't say "voices in your head." If you have those, you're reading the wrong book.) That voice I am referring to is you. It's the part of you that picks up on stuff. It's the area of your mind that processes that amazing gut database of experiences, faces, places, and things. They all come together to "speak" to you, and they are very often very right.

MEDITATE ON IT

If you're not a praying person or a meditating person, may I be blunt?

Become one.

It doesn't need a name. If you don't want to call it praying or meditating, call it whatever you want. Call it "sitting quietly and letting my mind rest." Call it "my time-out." Call it "contemplating my 'gut.'" It doesn't even need a name. For me, I call it praying. That's what works for me. If not for you, it's all good.

You have to listen to hear. To benefit from its message, you have to give the other voice, even if it's your own inner voice, the space and respect to speak.

Have you ever sat back and quietly watched someone trying to reason with, or worse, shout down a toddler having a tantrum? If you haven't, I highly recommend it. The entertainment value is awesome! It is hysterically funny to sit back and watch someone try to do this. (Unless it's your spouse. Trust me, that won't go over well.)

When I see this happen, I want to say to the adult in the scenario, "Do you really think that little kid, whose brain is barely past being a baby, can hear your voice no matter how loud you're screaming? Do you really think he can understand your psychobabble when he's in that electric, wild, out-of-control state?"

I know there are some experts who would disagree, and I'm certainly open to learning, but while in the process of raising two kids, one who is a toddler right now, and taking care of possibly thousands of kids over my pediatric nursing career, I've learned that the best thing to do is get them and you to a "quiet place."

When my kid has a meltdown in a restaurant because he hasn't had a nap and he's hungry and tired and now his red crayon broke, I don't allow him to scream himself red-faced while the other patrons are trying to eat their chicken salad sandwiches! I also don't sit there yelling at him or trying to have an intelligent, rational conversation with him. He's not rational right now! He's tired.

He's three!

I pick him up calmly and we walk outside. I don't do this angrily. I don't scare him. I don't get mad or get loud. That NEVER works. I let him do his thing, in a quiet place. I do what I can to calm him. When he is in a different state, then we talk. (I get great results with this. Call me "the toddler whisperer"!)

In a quiet place and in a different state, I correct him. I can now comfort him and teach him the rules of the road for restaurant behavior. This is how we roll in the Bluni house. It seems to work. Everyone says that he's a pleasure to go out to eat with.

I know everyone parents differently. But even if you disagree with me, please tell me you understand the point I am making. Can you see the image I am trying to create? Your mind is like that tantrum-throwing toddler. You can yell at it and threaten it and say really intellectual things to it, but until your mind is in a different state, until it has stopped freaking out, until you have shoved a banana in that monkey mind's mouth and he's quietly swinging from his happy tree, it won't have an impact at all.

If you strongly disagree with me, that's fine. If you are about to just flip out and lose it, then please step outside to calm yourself down. When you're calm, come back in and continue reading. (See, I got this down!)

So, do what works for you. Find some time to get quiet. Now unless you work in a library, museum, or at a cemetery, it can be hard to find quiet places at work. So this may have to happen on a day off or after work. If your home is quiet, then find a spot on your comfy couch and be quiet. (In full disclosure, I have a fun toddler and a teenager, who is getting really good at playing guitar, so my house is usually *not* my best option.) If you want to learn how to meditate, look up books on the subject or look for places in your city that teach it.

But for now, Grasshopper, let me show you how to at least start your journey to a quieter mind.

First, sit quietly. Don't force any thoughts. When they come, let them come. Then let them go. If you think, *Oh, I need to go to the store today to buy cheese*, think it and then let it go. Don't start thinking about what kind of cheese, or whether you have cheese coupons, or if you should even eat cheese because you're getting a little lactose intolerant. Then you start wondering if they have special cheese for lactose intolerant people and asking yourself if a cow can become lactose intolerant... AHHHHH! Been there. A lot. Think it, breathe through it, and let it go.

When you get to a point where you're not really having a million thoughts, you're getting "quiet." Like anything else, it takes practice, so don't get frustrated if this doesn't come easily to you in the beginning. Just do this with no other goal in mind. A lot of experts advise to just pay attention to your breath. (No, not how it smells. The rhythm of it!) Or listen to your heartbeat. Some people play meditation music. Do whatever works for you.

After a week or so of doing this for anywhere from 10-30 minutes a day, you'll learn how to get quiet. Then some cool stuff starts to happen.

You can use that time to ask yourself questions: Should I transfer to that new department? What do I think of Rich? Do I trust this potential new partner? Then, sitting there quietly and letting your thoughts kind of drift as you ask yourself an important question, often remarkable things will happen. You "hear" things. Your "gut" speaks to you.

When you picture that new position, you see a lightning flash, which you interpret as a bad thing. Where did that come from? Your gut is telling you something. When you question your trust for a new work associate, you may realize they look like an old flame who did you wrong! Oh, that's where that came from! Your gut is telling you that the only reason you have reservations about that person is because they look like your ex. So maybe you should give them another chance.

Are you going to see intense visions and hear angelic voices? Uh... maybe. But, honestly, and I'm sorry to say this, the odds are that you will not. Just being real with you.

Get Realizin'

However, what may happen is you get some clarity. You'll realize something. The origin of the word "realize" means to bring something into existence. So, the reality, the answer, the truth is brought into existence by your gut. It becomes real for you.

The next part of this is that since you're now more in tune with yourself, things start to become "realized" even when you are not doing your quiet exercise. You start to become a little more in tune with that gut.

Women call it "women's intuition."

You know what men call it?

"Men's intuition."

Sorry. Couldn't resist. Really though, tapping into your intuition starts to become a little more natural. I've met some truly successful people.

People who have excelled in business, finance, relationships, fitness, spiritual pursuits, and academics. When I look for similarities between these people, and there are several, one of them is that they trusted that small voice inside them. They made decisions, multimillion-dollar decisions, life or death decisions, based not only on their research and knowledge of the situation but also on what their gut told them.

Often we get really lost in the weeds at work because we don't know where to turn. We not only doubt others, we begin to doubt ourselves. Maybe you made a really bad call or choice in life, and it knocked you down. Join the club.

I'm not going to write about all of the amazingly successful people who have failed enormously before they succeeded, because that would be a huge book. Research anyone who you feel is a success. Chances are, if you do some real digging, you will learn that they failed at some point on their journey. Success, true success, isn't handed to anyone. Success isn't just earned. It is earned and given and taken away, multiple times.

So, maybe you failed once, or twice, or a lot. Good. You now know one or two or a lot of things to not do again! Those failures should not be used as excuses to never trust yourself again. Maybe you just need to work on listening to your gut. And that's okay.

There are many things that can lead us to being more engaged when it comes to work. While many of those things are "out there" for you to go get and bring back, even more of them are "in here" to retrieve and bring out of yourself. Your intuition is a tool you cannot do without. It comes from that deeper place. That wiser place. It can be the guiding light that gets you out of those dark places.

Get quiet when you can. Take time to allow that monkey mind of yours to take a time-out. Then listen to it. It has some amazing things to teach you.

CHAPTER
18

STRAWBERRY SHAKES

Knowing your "big reasons" leads you to achieve "big results."

Most of us got into our chosen field for "big reasons." For my healthcare, pastoral care, military, education, law enforcement/firefighter/EMT, stay-at-home parent, and social service friends, this may come into view very distinctly. For these folks, it was and is all about helping others. Making a difference.

Of course, many fields can be connected to these "big reasons." I just can't list them all here. But even if you aren't in one of these fields, I believe there is a big reason behind why you do what you do. For some it may be more obvious than others, but it is there for all of us.

Our "big reasons" are the reasons we do something that go beyond the obvious. Our "big reasons" are what keep us engaged. When a leader or an organization wants to talk about "employee engagement," the most important thing that they can do is immediately begin to look for and focus on their workers' "big reasons."

All of us want to make a living, but many of us go beyond that and we want to make sure that we have a life worth living, especially when it comes to our work. Your "big reasons" are the deeper drivers of what it is that you do. Some people connected with their "big reasons" at a very young age. For example, my beautiful wife, Dawn, has wanted to be a nurse since she was a little girl. Our friend Brian wanted to be a fire-fighter since he was a kid, and actually became one at an age when many of us were still clutching our high school diploma thinking, *Okay, now what?* Both of them live lives where it is abundantly clear that they are engaged with their "big reasons" for why it is that they do what they do and they're both amazing at their work.

For many, your "calling" came early. For some, it came much later. Many of you may be on what's often called a "second career." For example, I've known many nurses who started nursing school in their 50s! For many, that's the age when you start to see retirement on the horizon. But, trust me, the folks who choose to go back to school later in life have a "big reason" for doing it.

"BIG" TIME

Sometimes in the minutiae of our daily work tasks, we lose the big rea-son connection. Instead, we focus on the little reasons that we do what we do. Such as, "I need to pay my bills." Or, "This is just a job. I just need to survive here for 12 hours a day and go home." Or, "I'm too old to do anything else." Or, "I've already been here for 10 years, better the devil you know than one you don't."

If you've been saying those or similar things lately, it's all good. I can re-late. We *do* need to pay our bills. I get it. But, if you are doing this work, even if it's not your dream job, don't you think it serves you well to at least look for a "big reason"? Let's take an example.

Assume you are someone who has always been good with numbers. Math was fun for you. (I have heard there are such people.) You find yourself working in a hospital environment and you are involved in the budgeting and spending for the organization. You are the master of Excel spreadsheets. You are a wizard at moving money around. But lately you feel a little...blah. You know? It seems like the same old thing. You just aren't feeling like you're "doing" something. You know the little reasons you are there, but not the big ones. Where do you begin? Ask yourself these questions:

1. What would happen to the people who work here if someone wasn't ensuring that the bills were paid and the money was available for payroll? Would they be able to do their work? Help their patients? Be there for the community? Would they be able to take care of their families? Their homes? Pay their bills? Enjoy some fun vacations? Pay their own or their kids' medical expenses?

2. What would happen to the patients treated at the hospital? If I didn't ensure that we could pay our debt, buy new equipment, etc., what would happen to that sick child who needs our help to treat her cancer? How many lives have we saved by making sure that we can provide the funds to do breast cancer or prostate cancer screenings to under-served communities?

3. If my team and I weren't here, simply put, would someone die? If we didn't manage the money efficiently and weren't

good stewards of it, how many trauma patients wouldn't have survived because of our lack of funds to provide a top-of-the-line CT scanner or MRI?

These are some basic questions but what they point to is that whole trickle-down effect that we cannot deny exists in our work. If each part of the "engine" of your workplace can't do what it is supposed to do, it surely affects the others. If the Finance Department drops the ball, the organization can't pay its bills on time and credit might be harder to come by, thus decreasing your ability to upgrade equipment. Well, then, that affects the frontline folks because they have to then continue to work with second-rate stuff.

So, in a healthcare setting this means that when a sick six-month-old baby is brought in with an illness that requires a certain piece of equipment that the organization couldn't afford to buy, that child will either get less effective treatment or will have to be transported to another organization. This might mean a delay in care, or it could result in other negative consequences caused by the stress of the transport.

If an environmental worker doesn't do his job and clean your office correctly, you might say, "Big deal." But let's say the flu is going around. Cleaning isn't happening correctly because the environmental worker basically doesn't see the "big reason" for their work. Phones and doorknobs aren't being sanitized. Peter, in the cubicle next to you, demonstrates some questionable handwashing practices, and he has been sneezing and coughing all day.

Now the bug has spread throughout the department, resulting in you and two other key players becoming very ill and calling in sick. Unfortunately, that important advertising project you've all been working on together will have to wait, even though it may be the very thing the organization needs to sell more product to stay afloat. The project gets delayed, no biggie, right? Well, while you were out sick for a week, your competitor had a very similar idea, and on your way back to work still sniffling and achy, you see a big billboard with a very similar idea beaming down on you. Your competitor beat you to the punch. Now, their stuff outsells your stuff three quarters in a row, and 25 people are getting laid off in the department down the hall from yours.

Did all that happen just because someone failed to sanitize a doorknob? No. But, can you honestly tell me it didn't contribute? No way. It did. Maybe more than we can even realize.

There really is no unimportant job, only people who fail to see the importance of their work.

Big reasons equal big results. Basically every major book on improving business outcomes, results, sales, or personal excellence says this. Most of them probably say it in much more academic terms than I'm doing here, but it boils down to this: When you have a deep understanding and connection to your "big reasons," your outcomes, both personal and organizational, improve massively.

If you're a leader, a manager, a director, a VP, or a CEO and you don't know your "big reason," pay attention. You need to figure it out. Fast. Once you do, get those who report to you to figure out theirs. Fast. And so on down the line. When everyone knows their "big reasons," you'll see deep, sustainable results. One of those results is engagement.

Real engagement. In addition to telling your stories, it is the deeper meaning of why you do what you do that takes you and those around you from being "present" to being "engaged." When we connect to our "big reasons," when our organizations and leaders look for this and speak to these big reasons, that is when they begin to see "big results." Quite frankly, this also helps you distinguish between the people who are taking up space in your organization and the people who are taking the organization into outer space!

SHAKE THINGS UP

Sometimes our "big reasons" come to us as a result of a singular event. Something that smacks us on the head and says, "Here I am!" For many of us, something that happens at work suddenly opens our eyes and hearts. We glimpse that "big reason," maybe fleetingly, but it is there. That moment is a reminder, a touchstone, maybe it's even Heaven-sent, to show you your "big reason" bright and clear like a blanket of stars shining on a clear, crisp night.

I call these "strawberry shake moments." Here's why:

When I worked in the PICU taking care of very sick children, it wasn't uncommon to bond with these young heroes and their parents. One time, there was a kid named JJ, who was such a hero. He and his mom were wonderful. They were alone in the world with no siblings or father in the picture. JJ and I became buddies. He was around 14, and I was in my late twenties. He was a quiet kid but also very funny. In fact, he made me laugh every day.

JJ had a complicated G.I. illness that caused him to be in and out of the hospital often. He would have to be fed intravenously for long periods of time, completely unable to eat solid food. During one such stretch he was improving and they were moving him out of the ICU to the regular medical floor with orders to advance diet as tolerated. This is "hospital speak" for "You can start with clear liquids and move down the food chain to real stuff if you don't get sick!" He was thrilled. I helped move him to the floor, and the admitting nurse there was someone who, well...let's say wasn't the most "engaged" fellow.

That made me nervous. I volunteered to get JJ some food and start the ball rolling, but the receiving nurse assured me, JJ, and his mom that he would make sure all was well. As I was being rushed back to the ICU to admit a child from the OR, I had to trust this was going to happen. I ended up having an incredibly busy night and went home late.

The next morning when I came in, I beelined it to JJ's room. He and his mom were awake, and the first thing I noticed was the IV beeping. JJ was still being fed intravenously. I immediately worried that he hadn't done well with eating but found out otherwise. The nurse just "couldn't get to it," and JJ never got the chance to take in any food except for some juice. I was mad.

Long story short, I made sure that JJ got some food, and finally he was on the road to munchy town. During my lunch break, I came back to see JJ on the floor. He was doing better. I asked him if there was anything that he was craving. Without missing a beat, he and his mom spoke in unison, "A McDonald's strawberry shake!"

Well, it just so happened we had a McD's on campus, so I ran down there and bought TWO huge pink shake monstrosities and brought them up quickly so they wouldn't melt in the hot Miami sun. (Hey, he waited long enough; I figured two shakes were better than one!) You should have seen his face! It was like I walked in with pink liquid gold!

He savored those shakes. He even shared some with his mom. (That's love!)

It was a great day. One of the last few he had. After going home and coming back to the hospital a few more times during the next few months, JJ lost the battle he waged so bravely. He passed away in our PICU. I was holding his left hand and his mom was holding his right. I miss that kid. I am 45 years old, and I think about him to this day. My oldest son is 14 as I am writing this, and when I look at him I can't help but think of my buddy JJ who was the same age when he died. I am so glad I met JJ and his mom.

JJ's funeral was one of the only patient funerals I went to in those days. It was so painful to me that years later I still had dreams about it. He was a shining star whose light was dimmed way too soon.

Awhile later I was at work on a Friday, and I answered the phone. It was JJ's mom. It was great to hear her voice. She asked me if I was working that weekend, and since I was, she wondered if we could have lunch that Saturday if time permitted. We agreed to meet, and it just so happened that it was a quiet day. Rare but welcomed.

We were walking down the path towards "restaurant row" in our busy metropolis of a medical center, allowing the Miami sun to warm us, but after getting caught up on the latest news of our lives, she stopped walking. Turning to me she asked, "Do you know what today is?"

I answered, "Yes, Saturday the 22nd."

She smiled and shook her head sadly saying, "Yes, but today is also the one-year anniversary of JJ's death. It was a year ago today."

Had that much time really gone by? I hugged her and apologized. She said, "No need to be sorry. I just felt that I wanted to spend this day with you. It was what JJ would've wanted. He loved you. You were like a brother to him. He always said that to me. It was just you and me with him when he died. I was holding his right hand and you his left. I will never forget that day." Neither would I, I reassured her. She asked me if it would be okay if she picked the lunch spot. Of course, you know exactly where we went.

To McDonald's.

We must have been quite a sight that day. Two grown people, sitting in our booth, holding up our strawberry shakes in a toast to JJ. She drank a toast to her only son, who had taught her to live, to laugh, to love, to cry, and that life is beautiful no matter when and how it ends.

I drank to a young man who reminded me that we all have a responsibility to each other, especially in healthcare, and that each need, even a strawberry shake, can be the most important thing in the world at a given moment. He taught me that we all have that "strawberry shake moment" that stops us in our tracks and brings our big reasons clearly into focus.

I will never forget JJ. Who do you remember? What moment stopped you? What are your "big reasons" for what you do? People don't become or stay engaged for little reasons.

What was your "strawberry shake moment"? You owe it to yourself to remember it.

CHAPTER
19

ENGAGEMENT REQUIRES "INSULATION"

Ever notice that the insulation put in walls is often "fluffy"? That insulation, like engagement, protects you from the "cold," keeps you safe from the elements, and sustains you. For your well-being and safety, it is not enough to simply have a "stone wall" around you if it lets in the cold. Sometimes, in order to survive, you need that "fluffy stuff."

So there you have it. We've spent some time together talking about what some folks call "fluffy stuff."

Look around you. Look closely at your "work life" and your friends' and loved ones' work lives. What are you hearing? Are you hearing that people need more training? Are you hearing that people need more certifications? Well, there is nothing wrong with any of that, and certainly many people would benefit from better training or more certifications, but is a shortage of training, regulations, and certifications really what makes your work life a struggle at times?

Is it a lack of any of these things that leads to disengagement? Are these "hard" skills lacking in such numbers that they are leading to disengagement? While they could be contributors, I hope I've made a reasonable argument that they are not the main sources.

The fact of the matter is that people are hurting on a lot of levels today. They are fighting to survive both economically and spiritually. Forward-leaning organizations know that it is unwise to wait until the walls of the fortress are crumbling to add stronger bricks. You can have the hardest, strongest walls, but if you don't have enough of that "fluffy stuff" to insulate those walls, to block out the cold, and to keep in the warmth, you will be left with a strong fortress filled with ice-cold warriors who don't have the energy to lift their swords and fight another battle.

That's what we are seeing today. It's like the foolish pharaoh ignoring all of the plagues upon his people. Despite their suffering, he would not free the captives. After all, his "fortress walls" were still standing. He thought he could wait it out. He was wrong.

Yes, you need the "hard walls" to protect the fortress. But to sustain it and to keep your "warriors" in the battle, you also need the "fluffy stuff" to insulate it to make the environment healthy, warm, and safe.

Winning the "war of engagement" can no longer be done by simply building a higher and stronger "fortress." We cannot expect to simply win a "war of attrition," where only the strong survive and the only sign we've won is that the fortress is still standing at the end.

We all know what we're doing now is not working. Of what use is a mighty fortress if it is filled with freezing, starving, disengaged warriors? You and I win this "battle" when we not only keep the fortress standing but we also realize engagement is built, and sustained, by insulating our fortress from the cold. It is preventative medicine. It is wise...and yes, sometimes it is fluffy.

So now it is up to you to install some "fluffy stuff" insulation at your organization. Or at least, I hope that's what this book has inspired you to do.

We are all hungry for engagement. The very meaning of the word shows us it is about emotional involvement, connection, presence. These are, by their nature, fulfilling things, and we need more of them at work— heck, in life!

I hope over the next few months you and your organizations are judging less, being fearless, looking at and talking about what really matters. That you're willing to be uncomfortable, trusting your gut, kissing fewer frogs, dealing with psychic vampires, and drinking strawberry shakes while driving your yellow cars over speed bumps!

Get this done! Get your fortress insulated! Get yourself and your team engaged!

Get fluffy!

ACKNOWLEDGMENTS

I would like to lovingly thank and acknowledge the following, in no particular order but with respect and gratitude:

Quint Studer, first, for your friendship and support, and second, for the vision and focus you bring to healthcare. You have saved lives and careers. I am grateful to be a small part of what you have created.

BG Porter, thank you for your mentoring and encouragement. You've been a blessing and an inspiration.

Bekki Kennedy, for the great opportunity you've given me; Dottie DeHart, Lindsay Miller, all at DeHart & Company, Jamie Stewart, and Candace Edwards, for your hard work, guidance, empathy, and friendship. Thank you ALL so very, very much!

My dear friends: Alan and Gina, Jennifer and Peter, Tom and Karen, Brian and Heather, Tyler and Jason (Monkey Stomp!), Josh and Michelle, Mandy and Matt, Aimee and Ken, David and Jim, Jeff and Portia, Christopher and Laurie, Dan T., Lexi, Devin and Miss Jennifer, and all my friends at Florida Hospital, your love and support mean the world to me. We have awesome friends!

All of my family, especially my mom, Ann, who always believed, my dad, Jack, who never leaves my heart, and my mother-in-law, Vickie, for your love and spirit.

Fonda and Art, thanks for always being there for us.

Sheila Martin, I just love working with you. Mallory, Tasha, and Stephanie B., you rock!

Renee Barnett, you are just simply "all that"!

Pastor Joel Hunter and Father Julian Harris (1 Corinthians 13:13)

The entire Studer Group team, in Pensacola and around the country, you are my friends and colleagues and I love you all. Thank you for all you do and give.

To those who call healthcare their home and to all of those who work with passion and heart in their endeavors. You never cease to amaze and humble me.

Liz Jazwiec, a true friend, the real deal, and the sister I always wanted.

WANT TO FEEL EVEN MORE INSPIRED? DON'T MISS RICH BLUNI'S AWARD-WINNING FIRST BOOK!

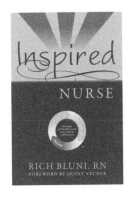 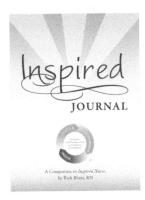

Remember your first day as a nurse? You thought, *What a privilege to do this work!*

It's true. Few other professions afford the opportunity to impact lives on such a profound level, not only physically but emotionally and spiritually as well. Yet the same qualities that make nursing so deeply rewarding can also make it a challenge, over time, to sustain your energy and passion. *Inspired Nurse*, along with its companion piece, *Inspired Journal*, helps us maintain and recapture those elusive qualities.

Rich Bluni, RN, reminds nurses and all healthcare employees why we chose this profession. He provides a wealth of action-oriented "spiritual stretches" that help us more fully integrate the gifts of nursing—joy, wonder, gratitude, insight, and grief—into our daily lives. What's more, his personal stories illuminate those sacred moments we all experience.

Bluni's books serve as a welcome validation that when we stay engaged and committed, we're more likely to provide extraordinary patient care in terms of both clinical outcomes and human compassion. Discover why they've inspired so many nurses—and so many healthcare professionals of all stripes—to reconnect to their passion and feel grateful for the profound difference they make in the lives of others.

To order *Inspired Nurse* and *Inspired Journal* at a special bulk discount rate, please visit www.firestarterpublishing.com or call 866-354-3473.

ADDITIONAL RESOURCES

About Studer Group:
Learn more about Studer Group by scanning the QR code with your mobile device or by visiting www.studergroup.com/about_studergroup/index.dot.

Studer Group˚ works with over 850 healthcare organizations in the U.S. and beyond, teaching them how to achieve, sustain, and accelerate exceptional clinical, operational, and financial outcomes. With the rapid changes occurring in healthcare due to the Patient Protection and Affordable Care Act ushering in the pay-for-performance era, this ability has never been more critical.

As the metrics our industry publicly reports get expanded—and as reimbursement is increasingly tied to these results—organizations are forced to get progressively better at providing top quality care with fewer dollars. Studer Group's unique and proven approach aligns goals, behaviors, and processes to create a sustainable culture of relentless consistency and quality care. The approach energizes and empowers healthcare organizations to successfully deliver their mission, impact margins, and ensure their ongoing success in this era of rapid change. This commitment to helping organizations accelerate their ability to execute led to Studer Group's receiving the 2010 Malcolm Baldrige National Quality Award.

Studer Group Coaching:
Learn more about Studer Group coaching by scanning the QR code with your mobile device or by visiting www.studergroup.com/coaching.

Healthcare Organization Coaching
As value-based purchasing changes the healthcare landscape forever, organizations need to execute quickly and consistently, achieve better outcomes across the board, and sustain improvements year after year. Studer Group's team of performance experts has hands-on experience in all aspects of achieving breakthrough results. They provide the strategic thinking, the Evidence-Based Leadership framework, the practical tactics, and the ongoing support to help our partners excel in this high-pressure environment. Our performance experts work with a variety of organizations, from academic medical centers to large healthcare systems to small rural hospitals.

Emergency Department Coaching
With public reporting of data coming in the future, healthcare organizations can no longer accept crowded Emergency Departments and long patient wait times. Our team of ED coach experts will partner with you to implement best practices, proven tools, and tactics using our Evidence-Based Leadership approach to improve results in the Emergency Department that stretch or impact across the entire organization. Key deliverables include improving flow, decreasing staff turnover, increasing employee, physician, and patient satisfaction, decreasing door-to-doctor times, reducing left without being seen rates, increasing upfront cash collections, and increasing patient volumes and revenue.

Physician Integration & Partnership Coaching
Physician integration is critical to an organization's ability to run smoothly and efficiently. Studer Group coaches diagnose how aligned physicians are with your mission and goals, train you on how to effectively provide performance feedback, and help physicians develop the skills they need to prevent burnout. The goal is to help physicians become engaged, enthusiastic partners in the truest sense of the word—which optimizes HCAHPS results and creates a better continuum of high-quality patient care.

Books: categorized by audience

Explore the Fire Starter Publishing website by scanning the QR code with your mobile device or by visiting www.firestarterpublishing.com.

<u>Senior Leaders & Physicians</u>

Leadership and Medicine—A book that makes sense of the complex challenges of healthcare and offers a wealth of practical advice to future generations, written by Floyd D. Loop, MD, former chief executive of the Cleveland Clinic (1989-2004).

Engaging Physicians: A Manual to Physician Partnership—A tactical and passionate roadmap for physician collaboration to generate organizational high performance, written by Stephen C. Beeson, MD.

Straight A Leadership: Alignment, Action, Accountability—A guide that will help you identify gaps in Alignment, Action, and Accountability, create a plan to fill them, and become a more resourceful, agile, high-performing organization, written by Quint Studer.

Excellence with an Edge: Practicing Medicine in a Competitive Environment—An insightful book that provides practical tools and techniques you need to know to have a solid grasp of the business side of making a living in healthcare, written by Michael T. Harris, MD.

Physicians
Practicing Excellence: A Physician's Manual to Exceptional Health Care—This book, written by Stephen C. Beeson, MD, is a brilliant guide to implementing physician leadership and behaviors that will create a high-performance workplace.

All Leaders
The Great Employee Handbook: Making Work and Life Better—This book is a valuable resource for employees at all levels who want to learn how to handle tough workplace situations—skills that normally come only from a lifetime of experience. Wall Street Journal bestselling author Quint Studer has pulled together the best insights gained from working with thousands of employees during his career.

Hey Cupcake! We Are ALL Leaders—Author Liz Jazwiec explains that we'll all eventually be called on to lead someone, whether it's a department, a shift, a project team, or a new employee. In her trademark slightly sarcastic (and hilarious) voice, she provides learned-the-hard-way insights that will benefit leaders in every industry and at every level.

The HCAHPS Handbook: Hardwire Your Hospital for Pay-for-Performance Success—A practical resource filled with actionable tips proven to help hospitals improve patient perception of care. Written by Quint Studer, Brian C. Robinson, and Karen Cook, RN.

Hardwiring Excellence—A BusinessWeek bestseller, this book is a road map to creating and sustaining a "Culture of Service and Operational Excellence" that drives bottom-line results. Written by Quint Studer.

Results That Last—A Wall Street Journal bestseller by Quint Studer that teaches leaders in every industry how to apply his tactics and strategies to their own organizations to build a corporate culture that consistently reaches and exceeds its goals.

Hardwiring Flow: Systems and Processes for Seamless Patient Care—Drs. Thom Mayer and Kirk Jensen delve into one of the most critical issues facing healthcare leaders today: patient flow.

Eat That Cookie!: Make Workplace Positivity Pay Off...For Individuals, Teams, and Organizations—Written by Liz Jazwiec, RN, this book is funny, inspiring, relatable, and is packed with realistic, down-to-earth tactics to infuse positivity into your culture.

"I'm Sorry to Hear That..." Real-Life Responses to Patients' 101 Most Common Complaints About Health Care—When you respond to a patient's complaint, you are responding to the patient's sense of helplessness and anxiety. The service recovery scripts offered in this book can help you recover a patient's confidence in you and your organization. Authored by Susan Keane Baker and Leslie Bank.

101 Answers to Questions Leaders Ask—By Quint Studer and Studer Group coaches, offers practical, prescriptive solutions to some of the many questions he's received from healthcare leaders around the country.

Over Our Heads: An Analogy on Healthcare, Good Intentions, and Unforeseen Consequences—This book, written by Rulon F. Stacey, PhD, FACHE, uses a grocery store analogy to illustrate how government intervention leads to economic crisis and eventually, collapse.

Nurse Leaders and Nurses
The Nurse Leader Handbook: The Art and Science of Nurse Leadership—
By Studer Group senior nursing and physician leaders from across the
country, is filled with knowledge that provides nurse leaders with a solid
foundation for success. It also serves as a reference they can revisit again
and again when they have questions or need a quick refresher course in
a particular area of the job.

Inspired Nurse and *Inspired Journal*—By Rich Bluni, RN, helps maintain and recapture the inspiration nurses felt at the start of their journey
with action-oriented "spiritual stretches" and stories that illuminate
those sacred moments we all experience.

Emergency Department Team
Advance Your Emergency Department: Leading in a New Era—As this
critical book asserts, world-class Emergency Departments don't follow.
They lead. Stephanie J. Baker, RN, CEN, MBA, Regina Shupe, RN,
MSN, CEN, and Dan Smith, MD, FACEP, share high-impact strategies
and tactics to help your ED get results more efficiently, effectively, and
collaboratively. Master them and you'll improve quality, exceed patient
expectations, and ultimately help the entire organization maintain and
grow its profit margin.

Excellence in the Emergency Department—A book by Stephanie Baker,
RN, CEN, MBA, is filled with proven, easy-to-implement, step-by-
step instructions that will help you move your Emergency Department
forward.

Institutes:

Learn more about Studer Group institutes by scanning the QR code with your mobile device or by visiting www.studergroup.com/institutes.

Taking You and Your Organization to the Next Level

At this two-day institute, leaders learn tactics proven to help them quickly move results in the most critical areas: HCAHPS, Core Measures, preventable readmissions, hospital-acquired conditions, and more. They walk away with a clear action plan that yields measurable improvement within 90 days. Even more important, they learn how to implement these tactics in the context of our Evidence-Based Leadership framework so they can execute quickly and consistently and sustain the results over time.

Excellence in the Emergency Department: Hardwiring Flow & Patient Experience

Crowded Emergency Departments and long patient wait times are no longer acceptable, especially with public reporting of data in the near future. We can predict with great accuracy when lulls and peak times will be, and we know exactly how to improve flow and provide better quality care. This institute will reveal a few simple, hard-hitting tactics that solve the most pressing ED problems and create better clinical quality and patient perception of care throughout the entire hospital stay.

<u>The Physician Partnership Institute: A Path to Alignment, Engagement and Integration</u>
The changes mandated by health reform make it clear: There will surely be some sort of "marriage" between hospitals and physicians. Regardless of what form it takes, we must start laying the groundwork for a rewarding partnership now. Learn our comprehensive methodology for getting physicians aligned with, engaged in, and committed to your organization so that everyone is working together to provide the best possible clinical care, improve HCAHPS results, increase patient loyalty, and gain market share.

<u>What's Right in Health Care®</u>
One of the largest healthcare peer-to-peer learning conferences in the nation, What's Right in Health Care brings organizations together to share ideas that have been proven to make healthcare better. Thousands of leaders attend this institute every year to network with their peers, to hear top industry experts speak, and to learn tactical best practices that allow them to accelerate and sustain performance.

<u>Excellence in Nursing</u>
Studer Group's newest institute, Excellence in Nursing, is dedicated to providing nurse leaders and their teams with the training and fundamentals needed to deliver quality patient-centered care. The daily challenges that nurse leaders face today require the right skills and tools to provide excellent care to our patients, while also managing operational priorities such as staffing, scheduling, and budgeting and the outcomes associated with them.

For information on Continuing Education Credits, visit www.studergroup.com/cmecredits.

ABOUT THE AUTHOR

Rich Bluni is a best-selling author of the books *Inspired Nurse* and *Inspired Journal* and a coauthor of *The Nurse Leader Handbook*, as well as a popular national healthcare presenter. Rich joined the Studer Group team in 2007 as an expert coach working with organizations all over the U.S. His clinical experience includes over 20 years in healthcare. Rich is a Registered Nurse and a Licensed Healthcare Risk Manager and has worked in Pediatric Oncology, Pediatric Intensive Care, Flight Nursing, and Trauma Intensive Care. Rich was an Emergency Department Manager as well as a Director of Risk Management and Patient Safety.

Rich is one of Studer Group's most sought-after keynote speakers for major healthcare conferences and seminars and has presented to tens of thousands of healthcare leaders, executives, and frontline staff at hundreds of healthcare organizations, hospitals, and medical practices in the United States and Canada. Rich is married to the love of his life, Dawn, who is also a Registered Nurse, and has two sons who make him smile every day, Rhett and Luke.

How to Order Additional Copies of

Oh No...Not More of That Fluffy Stuff!
The Power of Engagement

Orders may be placed:

Online at:
www.firestarterpublishing.com

Scan the QR code with your mobile device to order through
the Fire Starter Publishing website.

By phone at: 866-354-3473

By mail at: Fire Starter Publishing
913 Gulf Breeze Parkway, Suite 6
Gulf Breeze, FL 32561

Share this book with your team—and save!
Oh No...Not More of That Fluffy Stuff! is filled with valuable
information for staff members at every level. That's why we're
offering bulk discounts when you order multiple copies.
(The more you order, the more you save!)
For details, see www.firestarterpublishing.com.

Oh No...Not More of That Fluffy Stuff!
is also available at www.amazon.com.